"I couldn't wait to see what this book was about! Seriously! *Seriously Therapeutic Play* will appeal to those who are passionate about inviting others to grow through self-expression and exploration. Offering a learning-by-doing experience where our fingers unlock the power of metaphors is seriously creative. Bravo!"

Ken Gardner, MSc, R Psych (CPT-S), *senior faculty member and co-founder of the Rocky Mountain Play Therapy Institute, Alberta, Canada*

"My father, a bricklayer, always said how important the foundations are to create strong buildings. This book provides foundational knowledge to create, to construct, to communicate, to explore and to process therapeutic material through the magic of play. It is easy to read and is framed beautifully using the biopsychosocial lens and neuroscience to support the base and leads on towards therapeutic integration."

Judi Parson, PhD, *MA play therapy, BN RN, discipline leader, and senior lecturer in play therapy at Deakin University, Victoria, Australia*

"Klassen, Hamilton, and Peabody have created the first of two texts dedicated to the biological, psychological, social, and biopsychosocial components of LEGO® play. This book is a must have. Intended as a guidebook for the facilitator of play, this book deep dives into the why behind the therapeutic use of LEGO®. Knowing what you are doing and why are essential to facilitating mental health services and this book does not disappoint!"

Jessica Stone, PhD, RPT-S, *licensed psychologist in private practice, Colorado, USA, co-creator of the Virtual Sandtray App®©*

"This well-written, thoughtful book describes the biopsychosocial research behind *Seriously Therapeutic Play with LEGO®* and offers an integrated perspective to support practitioners in using this approach with their clients. I guarantee that after reading this book you will look at LEGO® bricks with a fresh perspective."

Lesia Shepel, PhD, RPT-S, *registered social worker in private practice, Manitoba, Canada*

"A must-read for anyone with LEGO® in their office, this book shares a profoundly impactful model as it describes the why behind a fascinating conceptualization of *Seriously Therapeutic Play with LEGO®*. Through the authors' invitation to play and the resulting journey through the exploration of emotional experiences via the metaphor of the bricks and the therapeutic powers of group and play therapies, this book brings the meaning of the model to life through personal and professional experiences."

Julie Nash, PhD, RPT-S, *licensed clinical psychologist at Riverside Psychological Associates, LLC, Connecticut, USA*

"The LSP facilitator in me needed to build a model in response to this book! Klassen, Hamilton, and Peabody provide a robust and comprehensive theoretical background to assist the reader in understanding the power of play using LEGO® as a medium for therapeutic interaction. The detailed practical case studies demonstrate a synthesised integration of the theory in practice to provide the reader with the stimulus to apply the knowledge for real-life situations."

Thomas Bevitt, MOT, *occupational therapy professional practice program convener/lecturer and course convener, University of Canberra, Australia*

SERIOUSLY THERAPEUTIC PLAY WITH LEGO®

LEGO® bricks are a staple in many child and play therapists' offices, and *Seriously Therapeutic Play with LEGO®* shows therapists and counsellors how to integrate LEGO® in a therapeutically valuable way. This book presents a therapeutic approach based in biological, psychological, and social research, one that supports participants as they build models that represent their thoughts, emotions, experiences, and reflections. Using a variety of evidence-based intervention techniques, chapters show clinicians how to incorporate the model and associated metaphors to help clients, and they do so in a way that is compatible with any number of therapeutic orientations or perspectives.

Though based in current research, *Seriously Therapeutic Play with LEGO®* is designed for psychologists, social workers, school counsellors, occupational therapists, clinical educators and supervisors, coaches, support workers, and other health care providers across the lifespan who wish to use play therapeutically.

Kristen Klassen, PhD, is a facilitator, trainer, and therapist who believes that play is at the core of all that we do and uses it to help others learn, grow, think, and be different.

Alec Hamilton, PhD, has been a practising psychologist with people of all ages for over 30 years, utilising positivity, joy, and playfulness to guide his clients and colleagues on their change journey.

Mary Anne Peabody, EdD, LCSW, RPT-S, is an associate professor at the University of Southern Maine and has published on adapting LEGO® Serious Play® in higher education, play therapy, and clinical supervision.

SERIOUSLY THERAPEUTIC PLAY WITH LEGO®

THE GUIDEBOOK FOR HELPING PROFESSIONALS

KRISTEN KLASSEN, ALEC HAMILTON AND MARY ANNE PEABODY

Routledge
Taylor & Francis Group

NEW YORK AND LONDON

Designed cover image: © Chequered Ink (font), Jaye Howard (cover design), and Janna Crerar (pictures)

First published 2024
by Routledge
605 Third Avenue, New York, NY 10158

and by Routledge
4 Park Square, Milton Park, Abingdon, Oxon, OX14 4RN

Routledge is an imprint of the Taylor & Francis Group, an informa business

ISBN: 978-1-032-19692-3 (hbk)
ISBN: 978-1-032-19693-0 (pbk)
ISBN: 978-1-003-26042-4 (ebk)

DOI: 10.4324/9781003260424

Typeset in Galliard
by Apex CoVantage, LLC

K.K. – *This book is dedicated to all of those who have played with me along this journey: Christopher, for being my constant, loving, and playful companion; Alec and Mary Anne, for playing with the words until they were right; and for all the clients and participants who bring their authentic, playful selves to my workshops and playroom.*

A.H. – *I want to firstly acknowledge the support and assistance given to me by my family, Anita, Will and El, Sam, Cooper and the inspiring twins A and S. Without my biggest critics, fans, and mentors, I would not have had the courage (or the time) to take on things like a book. Thank you, Kristen and Mary Anne, for being encouragers and supporters throughout the whole process; thanks for asking me to be a part of this endeavour; it has been fun. Finally, I must give a massive shout-out to my clients and students who teach me something new daily. I am so fortunate to have at my door young people who skip, laugh, fight, cry and play their way through life – living their lives to the full every day.*

M.A.P. – *I dedicate this to my family. First, my parents for promoting a love of learning; second, to my husband Glenn for always supporting my playful adventures; and third, to my children, Katie and Matt, who continue to be playful souls. Finally, to Abel, my grandson, whose very creative LEGO® creations and imaginative stories keep me young!*

CONTENTS

ABOUT THE AUTHORS

Kristen Klassen, *PhD, CCC:* Kristen comes from a strong academic background, crossing qualitative and quantitative fields, examining human development from a wide variety of contexts. She holds a PhD in applied health sciences, an MSc in disability studies, an MA in counselling psychology, and a BSc in kinesiology. In addition to teaching at the University level, she is certified to train new facilitators in the LEGO® SERIOUS PLAY® (LSP) method and has developed a post-foundation training using the methodology in the treatment of mental health conditions such as depression, anxiety, PTSD, chronic pain, and interpersonal challenges. She applies this unique skill set and knowledge background in her work as Certified Canadian Counsellor and as Play Therapist.

Alec Hamilton, *PhD, MAnalyPsych, MCouns, GradDipAppSCi, BEd, Reg Counselling Psychologist.* Alec is a practising psychologist with over 30 years of experience in private practice and schools. He is a Certified LEGO® Serious Play® (LSP) facilitator. Alec has also taught educational psychology, psychology, and counselling at Australian and Canadian universities. He is an evidence-based practitioner who focuses on the common factor in adapting his approach in working with his clients and views playfulness as a critical aspect of his approach to therapy. Alec has been an

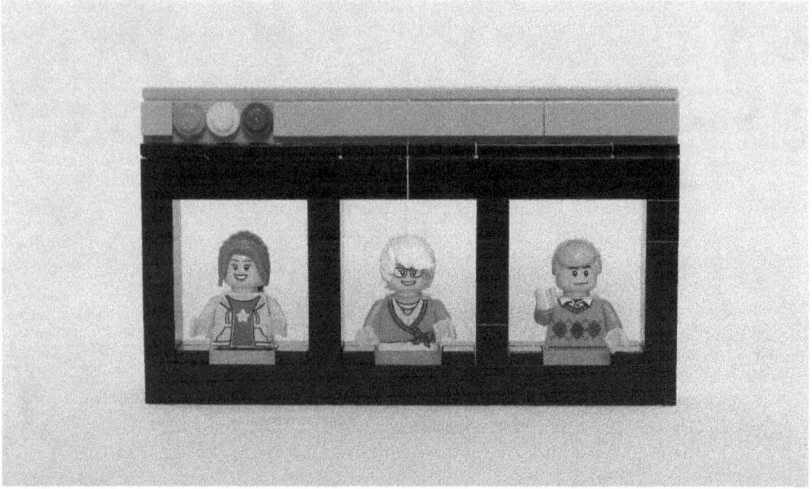

Figure 0.01 *A model illustrating the three authors as minifigures in Zoom panels.*

invited speaker on various topics, including brain functioning, parenting, child and adolescent development, and therapeutic presence.

Mary Anne Peabody, *EdD, LCSW, RPT-S:* Mary Anne is an associate professor, a licensed clinical social worker, a registered play therapy supervisor, and a certified LEGO® SERIOUS PLAY® facilitator. She has been a contributing author to several books on play therapy and has written numerous articles in peer-reviewed journals, including two publications on her LEGO® SERIOUS PLAY® research in higher education. She has presented nationally and internationally on adapting LEGO® SERIOUS PLAY® within play therapy venues.

Acknowledgements

A genuine and heartfelt thank you to Janna Crerar for generously sharing her photography skills (and for her endless patience with photographing LEGO® models!).

Introduction
Seriously therapeutic play

An introduction via
a biopsychosocial "lens"

Kristen Klassen, Mary Anne Peabody, and Alec Hamilton

Introduction

LEGO® bricks are a staple in many child and play therapist's offices. However, although many clinicians see the value of using a tool children naturally gravitate to and engage with, they struggle to integrate LEGO® in a therapeutically valuable way. Furthermore, many therapists who work with adults may be put off using a "child's toy" and struggle even to perceive the therapeutic value of the playful approach presented by the use of LEGO®.

The available literature to date is not of significant benefit; most available approaches to the use of LEGO® within the context of change are prescriptive and directive (such as LEGO®-based clubs, which focus on the "rules" of social relationships). These approaches do not necessarily resonate with the practitioner's natural approach or theoretical orientation. This book presents the foundations of our therapeutic approach to using LEGO® in a way that has depth, is flexible and adaptable, and is based on biological, psychological, and social research – i.e., from a biopsychosocial, integrative perspective.

While we conceptualised and developed this book in the context of play, we recognise that what we are proposing is not really play in the traditional sense. When we set out to articulate how we have been using

DOI: 10.4324/9781003260424-1

LEGO® within our professional practices, we saw that our "serious play" process allowed us to see the therapeutic world differently and interact with our participants in a very different way. Even though the three of us are in entirely different parts of the world and we practise with different theoretical orientations and diverse populations, we found a profound, shared experience in the "serious play" process – what we have called Seriously Therapeutic Play with LEGO® (STP).

We also debated long and hard whether this process should be called Seriously Therapeutic Play or Serious Therapeutic Play. The Oxford English Dictionary (Oxford Languages, 2023) primary definition of seriously is with "earnest intent," whereas the primary definition of serious is "solemn" or "grave." We also ultimately went with the adverb version, as it emphasises the therapeutic aspect of the approach.

This book is our guidebook to "why" we believe the therapeutic use of LEGO® is both valuable and an excellent resource in any therapist/ facilitator's tool bag. It is our foundational piece to STP. Following this, we plan to produce the playbook on the "how" of STP in practice, which will provide the reader with practical solutions and supporting materials.

Throughout the book, we have intentionally used the descriptor "facilitator," as we feel it captures a more diverse range of people working with others to promote change. The facilitator does not need to be a formally trained clinician; there are many ways of knowing. However, our core assumption is that the facilitator is in a professional relationship with another person or group to assist them in some way. The facilitator is in a role that takes on the responsibility of assisting others towards change. We believe many change efforts are therapeutic but not considered therapy. This is not to suggest that you don't require some background or training to be successful in using LEGO® in therapeutic interventions. We simply hope that this book is read by many people from diverse and wide-ranging fields of practice; people we haven't even thought of will use this approach in ways we never imagined!

Similarly, we have used the term "participant" or "client" instead of student or patient to describe those who we work with as it more accurately matches "facilitator". It also offers a broader perspective of the individuals and groups we assist in promoting and aiding change.

Our approach to using LEGO® in therapy, STP, centres around a relational approach, and, although we use the word "group" in some chapters, we accept that "group" may also be two people. Furthermore, we recognise this is a reciprocal process; the facilitator and participant contribute to the dynamic relationship required for change.

We firmly believe that everyone can benefit from play and gain value from the experience of playing. However, both play therapy and serious play mean something different than play. The definition of play includes an element of "purposelessness," with no requirement for learning objectives or intent for play to be valuable. Serious play is, however, inherently purposeful and goal-directed. To this end, we draw a strong distinction between playing with LEGO®, LEGO® SERIOUS PLAY®, and our Seriously Therapeutic Play approach.

If you are a sandtray therapist or use a sandplay approach, you may ask how STP differs from sandtray interventions. After all, both approaches provide specific metaphoric materials and direct prompts from the therapist, allowing sufficient time to create those metaphoric representations. Additionally, both approaches include a verbal processing phase where participants make meaning of their construction, and the therapist utilises careful processing skills to guide the participant in fully exploring the meaning of their creation. However, in sandtray, the miniatures and

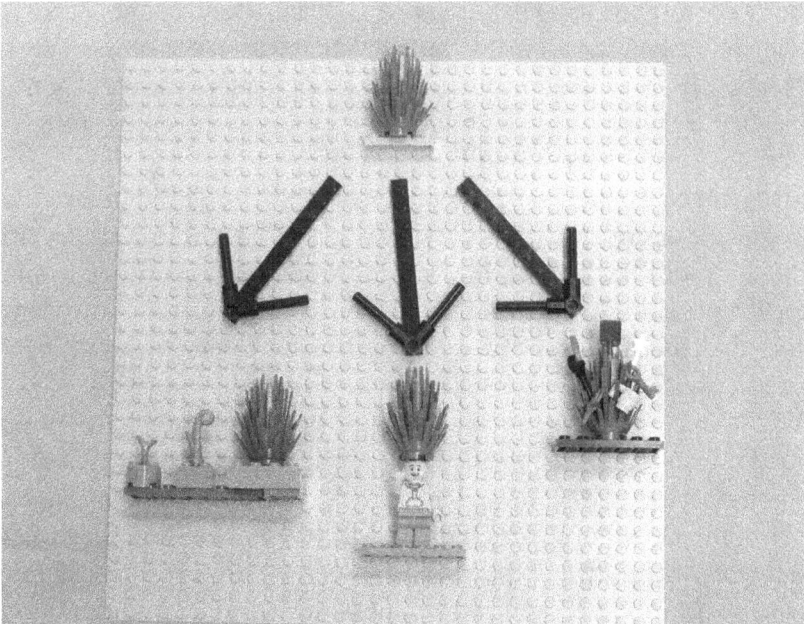

Figure 0.1 *A LEGO® model illustrating three different symbolic uses of the spiky green bush piece.*

objects used within the tray come imbued with meaning and symbolism. In contrast, LEGO® bricks have no meaning, allowing for creative, new, and original metaphors. Even pieces with some distinct symbolic characteristics (such as the spiky green bush piece, for example) can represent multiple metaphors (growth, a head exploding, divergent ideas, etc.).

In developing and sharing that meaning, "the [participant] must both build and create the story themselves, instead of being guided by the images elicited from the miniatures. [Participants] literally think through their fingers in a learning-by-doing experience that invites expression and deeper learning" (Peabody, 2015).

Furthermore, LEGO® in the therapeutic space navigates the line between permanence and impermanence in a way that the sandtray cannot. While the sand itself is impermanent and flows between built shapes and structures, the miniatures and objects used are permanent and cannot be altered meaningfully. By contrast, LEGO® models can be built, broken down, and rebuilt continuously.

Alternatively, if you are trained as an LSP facilitator, you may ask how the STP approach differs from the LSP process. Within an LSP workshop, past the individual build, the individual is first expected to self-regulate and then collaborate with the collective in building a more extensive construction. When using LEGO® in therapy, our purpose is to actually hold the individual (or the individual within the group), protect their space, facilitate their exploration process, explore the parts of themselves they are not seeing, and build their self-understanding through the constructed metaphor(s). Additionally, within an LSP workshop, affect is typically not centralised in the process, whereas in an STP approach, there is an explicit desire to focus on affect. Within STP, there is an invitation in the questions themselves to divest the emotional experience from the self and imbue it into the model, allowing the facilitator to investigate further that affective experience – in essence, broadening and deepening the participant's capacity for self-awareness and self-regulation.

With respect to the organisation of this book, we have roughly divided it into four parts; the first three chapters focus on the biological components; the middle three chapters focus on the psychological components; the next four focus on the social components; and the final two chapters are integrative of the biopsychosocial approach. These divisions are somewhat arbitrary, and you will notice an overlap of some concepts in the various sections. For example, we discuss how metaphor operates on a neuropsychological level, an individual psychological level, and a social level.

Chapter 1 takes the development of metaphor into the third dimension, in alignment with our brain structures and functions. Unlike most other strategies, STP shifts us out of the two-dimensional metaphor into a world that can be literally turned on its head! Perhaps for the first time, we can see things more clearly, helping us to understand positionality, perspective, and a view from another side. The physical 3-D representation of the LEGO® constructions takes us outside our language-based descriptions and into a simply constructed representation that develops as the bricks' click' into place. This opens up the possibility of emerging new metaphors that could not be seen within a 2-D representation or were previously unknown.

Chapter 2 investigates, from a neuropsychological perspective, how building, constructing, and thinking with our hands is therapeutic in itself and provides an opportunity for us to understand our world afresh. Using one's hands allows us to take information from the world without the necessity of conscious thought and allows the brain to "switch off" and process things more deeply. We can tap into things just below consciousness and facilitate problem-solving breakthroughs. Furthermore, using our hands is also often pleasurable just in itself.

Chapter 3 explores the innate, biological nature of play. We begin by defining play in rather clinical terms as voluntary, distinctive activity, often described as neither goal-directed nor rule-based. We then explore a little of the biology of play and how this information might help us further our understanding of the foundations of STP.

As noted, section 2 examines the psychological aspects of the biopsychosocial approach. Chapter 4 explores the psychological factors at play underpinning STP. We further our definition of play by examining play therapy and serious play and then discuss the psychological processes within STP that assist the individual to invest fully in the method and benefit therapeutically. These factors include the development of psychological safety through experiential methods, the experience of flow, the advantage of the common third, and therapeutic presence.

Chapter 5 looks at how language plays a crucial role in shaping interactions, both from the perspective of improving communication when we share a common language and hindering it when we fail to understand each other. This chapter investigates STP's capacity to overcome many of the limitations of spoken language and create a common language through a standard set of principles and strategies. These include actively "listening" to the model in its physical form, open-ended questioning and inquiry directed to the model, maintaining and deepening therapeutic metaphors, and prompting of storytelling or storymaking to help clients express themselves fully.

A key aspect of any therapeutic exchange is the development and understanding of one's story. However, theoretical orientations ascribe the "problem" differently, and this difference has led to often challenging conversations. Chapter 6 explores how we believe STP can illuminate the story within the context of a range of therapeutic approaches. We look at STP from the lens of psychoanalytic therapy, cognitive-behavioural therapy (CBT), person-centred therapy, narrative therapy, and solution-focussed therapy, as well as from a common-factors approach. The limitations of STP as an assessment technique are also explored.

The third section of this book dives into the social experience of this biopsychosocial intervention. Chapter 7 explores humans as social beings who are at the heart of every complex system, including our families, social groups, workplace relationships, community, and societal ecologies. At its basic level, a system is a group of interrelated, interacting, or interdependent parts that form a unified whole, working on a specific purpose. This is analogous to building with LEGO® bricks to create a three-dimensional model in response to a purposeful question. The dynamic experience of an STP group focuses more on the interplay between participants and the narrative stories, models, and challenges individuals and the group co-create.

In Chapter 8, we continue exploring how humans grow socially, emotionally, physically, intellectually, ethically, and expressively within networks of relationships. Borrowing from Bronfenbrenner's (1979) ecology model, we explore the interdependence and social complexities of our physical and mental health and why social engagement in play-based experiences matters to our overall well being. At the group level, we look at how STP assists in creating a dynamic multiplying effect between the facilitator's relationship with the group and the group members with one another. We explore the questions: why do we see accelerated group cohesion during STP? Why do these groups dive quite quickly into emotional expression? How does building with LEGO® and sharing with others help make social connections? The answers may lie in the social side of health.

At the heart of the LEGO® System of play is an "everything connects to everything else" notion, beginning with the brick's interconnecting studs and tube system. This mindset of a connecting system helps explain the social experience of STP, which encourages groups and individuals to think, build, and share.

We explore in Chapter 9 how the therapeutic powers of play connect with the group work factors to bring about change efforts. A brief review of the two different "factors of change" (Schaefer & Drewes, 2014; Yalom & Leszcz, 2020) will be shared, primarily focusing on the specific factors that most frequently arise in STP groups. These selected factors will help practitioners gain insight into the social nature of STP as a therapeutic application. We also capitalise on the functions of STP for providing awareness and skills for social and emotional learning and reflective practice. We share a model of reflective practice that fosters social skill development and presents an opportunity for new knowledge and social connections.

In Chapter 10, we explore how the theories of social constructivism and constructionism (particularly relational constructionism) help us to understand how knowledge is created through language-rich interactions within a relationship. By providing serious play opportunities in therapeutic and non-therapeutic settings, we can help participants elicit emotional responses that drive learning and new understandings. We have found that, when the STP process moves from individual to shared model building, the experience becomes broader and more profound. Therefore, we explore the broaden-and-build theory (Fredrickson, 2004) that states positive emotions broaden our thoughts and actions (e.g., to explore and seek, to be creative, and to savour life experiences), which consequently builds personal resources (e.g., psychological well being).

The final section of this book brings all our discussions and ponderings together in a practical and meaningful way. Chapter 11 is less academic and draws on our personal experiences. We present several case studies illustrating how we have implemented the STP strategies in various therapeutic contexts. From individual therapy to group therapy (both virtual and in-person) to families and couples to supervision, current methodology implementations are detailed. Quotes and pictorial examples from facilitators and participants alike express how not only the 3-D nature of the bricks but also the dynamism of the approach allows us to see what "jumps out," "what's now there that wasn't there before," and "what your hands have expressed that your words didn't."

The final chapter provides some fundamental tenets to integrating LEGO® successfully into therapeutic practice. We have drawn from our experiences and present both best practices that have worked for us and consistently bring positive results and the lessons learnt through trial and error (i.e., those practices that, in our experience, do not bring about successful outcomes). This chapter serves as an overview of the accompanying playbook and highlights some key learning points for therapeutic facilitators who wish to engage in the training.

At its core, the Seriously Therapeutic Play with LEGO® (STP) approach is designed to support participants in articulating their life stories through the construction of LEGO® builds. Participants use metaphors to describe and assign meaning to components of their models to amplify their understanding of their reflections. Facilitators from any number of therapeutic orientations or perspectives can utilise the participants' builds and associated metaphors to help progress their change journey and engage new life stories. These builds, we have found to have successfully represented our participants' thoughts, emotions, experiences, and reflections and offered new insights. In the words of one participant, "some models speak to you in a way that words cannot." We hope this book supports you in your practice of helping others change using play.

References

Bronfenbrenner, U. (1979). *The ecology of human development: Experiments by nature and design.* Harvard University Press.

Fredrickson, B. L. (2004). The broaden-and-build theory of positive emotions. *Philosophical Transactions of the Royal Society of London: Series B, Biological Sciences, 359*(1449), 1367–1378. https://doi.org/10.1098/rstb.2004.1512

Oxford Languages. (2023). *Seriously definition.* https://tinyurl.com/mr3hr4cy

Peabody, M. A. (2015). Building with purpose: Using LEGO® SERIOUS PLAY® in play therapy supervision. *International Journal of Play Therapy, 24*(1), 30–40. https://doi.org/10.1037/a0038607

Schaefer, C. E., & Drewes, A. A. (Eds.). (2014). *The therapeutic powers of play: 20 core agents of change* (2nd ed.). John Wiley & Sons.

Yalom, I. D., & Leszcz, M. (2020). *The theory and practice of group psychotherapy* (6th ed.). Basic Books.

CHAPTER 1
LEGO® AS A 3-DIMENSIONAL TOOL

Alec Hamilton

I started my professional journey as a teacher. Perhaps surprisingly for my teachers, I taught maths. Maths was not something I loved, nor was I particularly good. I loved biology, psychology, and environmental science but had to take several maths units to get the degree. After the first year of classes focusing on high school maths, I realised my limitations and decided to try some primary school maths. I discovered maths was way more interesting when you used your hands. It was easier to understand when you could manipulate things in space and "see" what you were doing. I graduated and moved to the country, and because I had maths on my CV, I was thrown into the deep end of upper high school maths. I worked one lesson ahead of the students, with my fantastic colleague Craig tutoring and helping me stay one step ahead – most of the time. In my second year of teaching, I moved to year ten and junior high school maths, to the students' relief. I had an opportunity, at this time, to join an innovative maths program, "RIME: Reality in Maths Education" (Lovitt & Lowe, 1984), which was alternatively titled "Making sum-think happen." The program called for "a radically different form of teaching and learning that makes more (and different) intellectual demands on the learner than conventional lessons and puts the teacher in a position of director of inquiry rather than information giver"

DOI: 10.4324/9781003260424-2

(Lampert, 1988). Problem construction and problem-solving became the focus, and the students started to do the thinking. The structure and underlying belief of the program were not to provide a set of instructions but rather resources to assist the class in exploring their world. I became a facilitator of learning, helping the students explore their world mathematically. We worked out "what to do when we did not know what to do," and the students became problem-solvers rather than information collectors. Problem-solving remains at the core of the Australian Mathematics curriculum today (ACARA, 2022).

How does all this relate to Seriously Therapeutic Play with LEGO® (STP)? This chapter explores how using our eyes – and hands – to manipulate things impacts our attention systems and our perception of the world, thereby facilitating our problem-construction and problem-solving abilities. Growth in therapy and during STP requires the perception of something outside ourselves, and through our perception, we can develop an understanding of the world and then build new learning. We first focus on "why" building with a manipulative like LEGO® helps our attention systems make sense of the world and develop our understanding of it. We then explore the "why" of building with LEGO® and how using 3-D imagery provides new perspectives, understanding, and learning.

Why build?: using our eyes and our hands in learning

It might be helpful to place some boundaries around the following discussions at the outset. There are several "neuromyths" (Dekker et al., 2012) surrounding using one's hands (or body) for learning. Those in education will be familiar with the push to have learning focussed and based on an individual's learning style – visual, auditory, or kinaesthetic (VAK). However, while information taken in via visual, auditory, or kinaesthetic modes may be processed in different brain areas, there is significant activation and transfer of information between these sensory modalities. It is an incorrect assumption that only one sensory modality operates at any given time. We are, therefore, proposing that, unlike some other approaches, LEGO® allows us to tap into a given mode at any given time. Through LEGO®, we can visually, auditorily, or kinaesthetically perceive our environment. However, learning and problem-solving require more than just perception; we need to be able to interpret the input of our senses and give this input meaning (OECD, n.d.-a). We can only construct our knowledge of the world through our endeavours to find meaning and understanding. This is the premise behind STP – the construction of meaning.

A second neuromyth is the duality of left- and right-brained learners: an individual is a right-brain thinker – creative, emotional, and artistic; or left-brained – rational, analytical, and logical. While some brain functions do occur laterally, individuals generally do not have a stronger side of the brain (Nielsen et al., 2013). "While there are some functional asymmetries, the two brain hemispheres do not work in isolation, but rather together in every cognitive task" (OECD, n.d.-b), highlighting that the brain is a complex interconnected system.

We probably don't have to mention the final neuromyth, but just in case, this one involves neurosexism: "men and women have different brains." Let us clarify: "modern neuroscientists have identified no decisive, category-defining differences between the brains of men and women" (Eliot, 2019, p. 453; Eliot et al., 2021). While differences in brain structure have been noted, most studies report correlational connections rather than causal ones, and brain structure is only one factor explaining behavioural sex differences. We must also recognise that individual differences are often more significant than identified sex differences (van Eijk et al., 2021).

The eyes have it

From birth, our brains learn how to construct and process in three dimensions. The human brain processes images faster than it does language. In a summary discussion of the research, Dunn (2021, para 2) indicates that "images are processed between 6 and 600 times faster" than word or sentence recognition. Complex narratives provide important information, which is where images come into their own, and 3-D constructions more so. Images can be processed more quickly than simple or complex language-based information. For example, researchers indicate that "more than 50% of the cortex is devoted to processing visual information." (Hagen, 2012, p. 35) and that we process and make meaning from them very quickly: "the meaning of an image can be extracted even when an image is mixed up in a sequence of six or even 12 images presented at 13 milliseconds per image" (Thrope cited in Trafton, 2014, para 13). However, visual processing is only part of the picture; we also need to take information in through our other senses, like touch, to make meaning of our experiences.

It is more than just the eyes: handy solutions and manipulatives

Gauntlett (2018) suggests that thinking and making are aspects of the same process; they connect thoughts, feelings, ideas, problems, solutions, and people. While not directly describing STP, he excellently articulates the process we observe in therapy:

> [Making] gets the brain firing in different ways and can generate insights which would most likely not have emerged through directed conversation. . . . Typically, people mess around with materials, select things, experimentally put parts together, rearrange, play, throw bits away, and generally manipulate the thing in question until it approaches something that seems to communicate meanings in a satisfying manner. Having an image or physical object to present and discuss enabled them to communicate and connect with other people more directly.

Drawing and painting can create static objects visually representing structures, relationships, or processes (Quillin & Thomas, 2015, p. 2). These creations can help improve student learning (Schmidgall et al., 2020) and have also been found to help define and build a business culture and describe and facilitate an awareness of the dynamic nature of relationships (Huff & Jenkins, 2002). Using our hands assists us in expressing our thoughts, making our ideas explicit, and facilitating one's understanding through visualisation and representation. Engaging our hands in building allows us to externalise our thoughts, feelings, and experiences to reflect and make meaning. The experience of creating with our hands helps the brain work from a different perspective and can generate insights not otherwise articulated through conversation (Gauntlett, 2018).

Manipulatives are physical tools like coins, pens, blocks, puzzles, paints, etc., that we can play with physically. They help us to engage and assist us to "make," often described as constructivist or constructionist learning. Both constructivism and constructionism are learning theories that have influenced educational psychology for decades (see Chapters 4 and 10 for further discussion). These theories contend that we construct knowledge best by experience and that our environment and the context it provides are central determinants of learning quality. A modern take on manipulatives (Willingham, 2017) suggests that they help us to understand and integrate new concepts. Because manipulatives can act as a metaphor, they can assist us in shifting our perspective and understanding of a concept and allow us to see things in more detail and build new meanings.

In her recent book (2021) and website (2021), Annie Paul presents fantastic research about thinking outside the brain via manipulatives. Paul suggests that material objects are helpful in that they seize attention, relieve the cognitive load, engage multiple senses, promote shared understanding, elicit gestures, and generate interactivity. While Paul's research is relatively new, Sarah Kuhn has been able to reiterate it in her practice (2022). We will discuss each of these in the following sections.

Seizing attention

Introducing the novel and the different creates situations that promote increased attention. In STP, we ask the participant to build a LEGO® model of the situation they wish to explore to assist in seizing attention. In my practice with young children and adults, I use the LEGO® Serious Play® (LSP) starter kit. I indicate that the box contains adult, serious LEGO®. It does not have a set of instructions for any set build but rather a range of different bricks they can use to build. The box is full of surprises, as the variety of bricks is generally unexpected. Those familiar with the kit frequently say, "I did not see this piece last time." Then I ask them to build, explaining that we will talk about the various features of the build once they are finished. As discussed in Chapters 5 and 10, the aim is to have the participant develop a narrative – or metaphor – around the construction. This will allow us to explore the various features of the build, looking for novel, surprising, or fresh aspects that the participant has not seen or seen in "that way" before.

The neuropsychology behind the STP process is linked to three theoretical constructs: the Markov blanket, the free energy principle (FEP), and the Bayesian brain. Each is discussed in detail below.

The Markov Blanket

The Markov Blanket construct pertains to a self-organising system with two aspects: the *sensory states* that do not influence the external but influence the internal; and the *active states* that influence the external and are dependent on the internal. There is conditional independence between internal and external states. The blanket is the "structure" created by conditional dependence. Hipólito et al. (2021) provide a visual depiction of the Markov Blanket in the context of the DMN and TPN. The *sensory states* can be viewed as the information we take in from our environment via our senses – the external influencing the internal. An *active state* might be our behaviour – how we interact with the world and characterise the internal affecting the external (see Friston, 2016).

The Free Energy Principle

Self-organising systems with a Markov Blanket will engage in behaviour that strives to minimise free energy. The movement of sensory input and action output operates to reduce the amount of free energy – the Free Energy Principle (FEP). FEP arises from statistical physics and is rather complex to discuss here. In simple terms, the principle proposes that biological systems like Neural Networks (see Isomura et al., 2022) are self-organising systems that work to reduce their "energy" costs and maintain their current state while operating in a constantly changing environment. The system is trying to work as efficiently as possible using the least amount of energy it can.

FEP states that any self-organising system must maximise the evidence for its existence, which means it must minimise any free energy by applying the existing model to any input from sensory states. The more the sensory input matches the brain's model of the world, the less free energy. FEP attempts to explain why a system might try to reduce the difference between the inputs, perception, and world model. The self-organising system selectively interacts with the environment to minimise the free energy (Hipólito et al., 2021) – i.e., it picks and chooses the input it processes to match its internal view of the world.

The Bayesian Brain

Connecting to FEP is the notion of the Bayesian Brain. The Bayesian Brain metaphor proposes that the brain actively creates explanations for its own sampling of the world. The brain oversees information gathering; it chooses which information to take in and which to exclude. The brain matches the data it collects with its worldview and then explains and provides evidence for its predictions of the world based on the information it has gathered. In other words, it utilises the FEP to maintain itself: selectively choosing information that produces less free energy – i.e., information that matches its current worldview.

To paraphrase the earlier section, our brain is a self-organising system with finite energy reserves. In the past, these energy reserves have been used to create a model of the world. This model is now used to evaluate information from our senses and referenced to our model. The brain wants to conserve energy and work as efficiently as possible, matching what comes in with what it already knows. Things outside what it knows or expects create a problem – free energy – as this new data requires altering the current worldview. Therefore, on occasions, the brain will choose not to fully or accurately sense something outside its worldview and process the input *as if* it matched the view it expected. A simple and dramatic example of this is the selective attention test, sometimes known as the gorilla experiment (Chabris & Simons, 2011). I will not give away the details here, but the experiment illustrates how the brain cannot see what is right in front of it. Three other videos developed by Manassi and Whitney (2022) and examples by Banaji and Greenwald (2016) also demonstrate how the brain's "old world" mental maps play with our perception.

To explain this further, we need to link to Chapters 2 and 3 and the role of the Default Mode Network (DMN) as a predictor: taking information from the past and creating future predictions. In terms that, perhaps, oversimplify things, the DMN is an internally focussed network influenced by sensory input, creating one's world model – *the sensory state*. The Salience Network's (SN) role mediates between external and internal stimuli, providing information for the DMN to build a dynamic world model. Interestingly, this is the same function attributed by Freud to the ego (Cieri & Esposito, 2019). The DMN makes "top-down" predictions based on the past; it tells us how things fit and what to think. The role of the Task Positive Network (TPN) (SN and frontoparietal network [FPN]) is to notice and explore the external world. Activation of SN increases connectivity between the DMN and the FPN, with SN providing the mechanism by which the attention can be switched on or off. The SN is involved in the bottom-up direction of salient events, detecting, integrating, and filtering relevant interoceptive, autonomic, and emotional information. It plays a crucial role in modulating and switching in and out of the DMN – *active state*. The research leads us to propose that the SN does *not* notice the unexpected – the different. In the earlier experiments, the input the DMN receives does not match the view held, producing a challenge requiring altering that view. Change requires energy – i.e., it would create free energy.

How STP grasps attention

The brain-body-hand connection is central to our understanding of working with STP. Our constructions help us smoothly flow from the external world to the internal world and back again. We believe and see from our participant experiences that building with LEGO® in STP allows us to notice the new, the novel, and the unexpected. From the perspective of the FEP, seeing things differently is expensive. The introduction of playing with LEGO® facilitates surprise, which "decouples" (Holmes & Nolte, 2019) the top-down/bottom-up interaction. The LEGO® build helps the SN and FPN to notice different things and perspectives through surprise. In essence, we trick our brains into seeing things differently, despite the cost of the new information. The DMN shifts into action in the background, acting as a creative predictor and planner. Research indicates that the DMN is active before and during spontaneous, creative thought and narrative production. The DMN can notice "conceptual variability" with the network, cuing the activation of different "conceptually disconnected (but contextually connected) mental states" (Christoff et al., 2016, p. 724). Being active in goal-directed thinking, building with LEGO® allows the brain to unconsciously slip back into the DMN and create "aha" moments (Laber-Warren, 2022), which also opens the opportunity for the DMN to reconfigure its worldview.

In therapeutic terms, using LEGO® facilitates the process by which the facilitator can help the participant shift out of their predicted habitual patterns, seizing the participant's attention and focusing on new views and perhaps creating "aha" or "eureka" moments. Using our hands to build allows us to take information from the world differently and work and explore without the conscious brain driving things. We see things afresh. We can tap into parts of our creativity and awareness outside verbal consciousness, outside our current internal worldview, and facilitate breakthroughs in problem-solving.

Relieving cognitive load

Cognitive load theory assumes that learning is a process that takes cognitive energy and is limited by the individual's working memory capacity. The brain's working memory can only take in small amounts of new information. Using knowledge already gained to obtain further knowledge reduces the energy required to assimilate any new information. If the information has been stored in long-term memory, then larger quantities of new information can be processed. The data already contained in our existing worldview does not produce as much free energy. The DMN can utilise its current worldview to process and accommodate the new, incoming information. We can also assist our working memory and cognitive load by employing various strategies. The strategy relevant here is the use of manipulatives, building with LEGO®. When new information is experienced, parts of the DMN become activated as changes to worldview might need to occur – i.e., during high cognitive load and challenging task-positive activities. Smallwood et al. (2013, p. 6) indicate that the DMN is utilised for "narrative comprehension," and when the integrity of the DMN worldview is maintained, "better task performance" occurs. Smallwood et al. also report that greater focus occurs if better coupling between the DMN and TPN occurs. There is a better match between internal and external worldviews in these situations.

The interplay between cognitive load and brain networks is complex, and research is emerging. However, some encouraging studies appear to explain how building with LEGO® might be assisting us to see afresh. For example, Jenkins (2019, p. 532) reports that "typical cognitive load tasks might inhibit processes of self-reflection, mental state attribution, or imagination with which the DMN is associated." However, Stuyck et al. (2022) report that cognitive load does not constrain "aha" experiences, allowing the mind to wander while completing a task-positive action allows insightful "aha" ideas to emerge. From this research, we conclude that building with LEGO® may help decrease cognitive load and shift away from the limits of one's current worldview, facilitating the SN to switch backwards and forwards between DMN and TPN, thereby developing and creating opportunities for new and novel understandings to emerge.

Promote shared understanding

A core aspect of LSP is using the LEGO® build to assist communication and develop a shared understanding of an issue or concept (Barton & James, 2017). To explain how STP helps in promoting the participants' and facilitator's shared understanding is illustrated in the following case example. When participants struggle with peer relationships, I often ask them to describe their friendship group in words, draw a diagram, or build a LEGO® model. An example is provided in detail in Chapter 11.

Verbally, the participant might explain in simple sentences, adding more information as they draw the connections between the individuals. The participants often report that drawing is more helpful than a verbal explanation as the complexity of the relationships becomes more evident in their picture. They can see how far apart or connected they feel and how far apart or connected the others in the group seem. They can spatially represent in two dimensions how the relationships seem to them. By adding colour links, we can see the specific connections as they view things now. We can also use this diagram to reflect on how the relationships may have developed since implementing an intervention. However, things start to emerge as we shift to building in 3-D with LEGO® and the participant's understanding deepens and things not previously noticed become more apparent. The LEGO® build assists the facilitator and participant in exploring the relationships at a greater depth than was possible before.

Elicit gestures

One of the cornerstone components of the LSP method is the gesture of "leaning in." Kristiansen and Rasmussen (2014), in their description and explanation of LSP, highlight what they describe as the 80/20 meeting culture.

> One or two individuals, often the most senior member and/or the meeting's host, control and enjoy the meeting. These 20 per cent of the participants take 80 per cent of the time, hence the title of 20/80. To make matters worse, these individuals typically contribute only 70 to 80 per cent of their full potential to solve the meeting's issues. The remaining 80 per cent of the participants contribute far less.
>
> (p. 16)

The LSP facilitator aims to create a different environment that involves the group "leaning in." In the 80/20 situation, most participants are mentally leaning out rather than engaging in the conversation. The "leaning in" environment sets up the opportunity for a 100/100 environment with all participants actively engaged fully. By participating in or observing an LSP workshop, you can see and experience the physical and emotional moment the group starts to lean in. Focus shifts from the individuals or the other participants to the concepts represented by the models in front of them.

In the therapeutic context, "leaning in" became part of the vernacular of counselling when Gerard Egan first published his book *The Skilled Helper* in 1975. Other comparative models have proposed similar strategies (Stickley, 2011). However, none have stood the test of time like Egan's model, now in its 11th edition (Egan & Reese, 2018). Egan's SOLER model trains beginning counsellors in nonverbal communication and how to be physically present with a participant. I was taught the skills in my early training and have successfully used the model to teach counselling students in Australia and Canada. The acronym stands for:

S   Face the person **S**quarely
O   Adopt an **O**pen posture
L   **L**ean in toward the person
E   Maintain **E**ye contact
R   Focus on being **R**elaxed

The SOLER process helps in counselling in two ways. Firstly, the body gestures in SOLER communicate that the facilitator is interested and engaged. Secondly, by modelling specific behaviour, we can trigger mirroring behaviour in another. Mirroring or mimicry "facilitate[s] emotional understanding and empathy . . . [and] increases social connections by creating social bonds" (Salazar Kämpf et al., 2021). During STP, the facilitator leans into the model and focuses on the model rather than the individual. This, in turn, leads to the participant leaning into their model and building engagement with the metaphor they created. Leaning in facilitates therapeutic presence, increasing empathy and social connection. When the participant and facilitator are attuned to each other and the model, this helps "to play a role in resolving ruptures and fostering exploration and the creation of new meanings" (Avdi & Seikkula, 2019, p. 217). Leaning in takes the eyes off the individual and onto the model, reducing eye contact, which some participants find stressful. My experience is that both young children, adolescents, and adults like the shift in focus; it helps establish the therapeutic alliance and gives the participant a sense of safety (for a deeper discussion of therapeutic presence and psychological safety, refer to Chapter 4).

Generate interactivity

Paul (2021, p. 157) describes generating interactivity as "the physical manipulation of tactile objects [which act] as an aide to solving abstract problems." The process of thinking and creating with LEGO® helps the participant develop a more complex understanding as represented by the object and the metaphor they create. The construction of the LEGO® metaphor captures what Schön (1993, p. 137) describes as a "generative metaphor": "a certain kind of product – a perspective or framework . . . and a certain kind of process – a process in which new perspectives . . . come into existence." When we develop generative metaphors, we create the capacity to see the unusual, the new, or the unknown, imbuing our thoughts and feelings with significance beyond any literal description, drawing us into comparison, and presenting the potential for new options for decisions and action. When communication involves metaphor, "the load on the intention recognition mechanisms increases, . . . invoking the involvement of at least some sub-parts of the mind-reading system [Theory of Mind]" (Bambini et al., 2011, p. 205). In essence, the physical metaphor constructed in LEGO® helps to facilitate recognition of communication and social interaction.

The generative nature of the LEGO® build highlights seen and unseen interactivity and reflects the switching mechanism operating between the DMN and TPN via a switching process within the salience network [SN] (Beaty et al., 2014, p. 163). The DMN plays a crucial role in perspective-taking and building a Theory of Mind (the ability to think about one's own and another's mental state), essential for comprehending nonliteral stimuli like metaphors (Rapp et al., 2012, p. 607). (See Chapter 2 for more details about DMN, TPN, and Theory of Mind and Chapters 5 and 9, which explore the importance of metaphor.)

Interactivity has many forms

Recently, an 8-year-old I was working with built what I thought was a very complex model. I asked them to explain what they were building. At that moment, they started to pull the model apart and throw the bricks into the box, along with sound effects of crashing and explosions and the noise of the bricks hitting each other. There was more joy on their face during this phase of the session than during the building. Pulling apart and making noise and the apparent pleasure of this process seemed significant. They had not previously taken a build apart during the session; they always left it for the next time. When they returned, they would ask if they could build something different, slowly and quietly pulling the old model apart, often asking for my help and chatting about general things that they were interested in at the moment. I realised from this experience that interactivity and value are not only in the construction – adding bricks – but also in the destruction – taking bricks away.

The work of Adams and Koltz (Adams et al., 2021; Kwon, 2021) highlights the importance of noticing different forms of interactivity. Leidy Klotz, an engineer, was using LEGO® to build with his child. They were building a bridge, and one leg – the side of the bridge – was longer than the other. Klotz turned around to get a new brick to add to the short side of the bridge; meanwhile, his child had simply removed a brick from the long side of the bridge. This prompted Klotz and Adams to investigate why people choose additive solutions and overlook subtraction as a problem-solving method. In their discussion of the research, they reference the development of balance bikes – two-wheeler bikes with peddles removed – as a great example of a modern innovation demonstrating the subtraction principle. Learning to ride a bike using trainer wheels – i.e., adding two support wheels – was the norm. Recent research (Mercê et al., 2022) has demonstrated that balance bikes increase a child's (and adult's) ability to ride by 2 to 3 years. Why did it take so long to move to balance bikes? "Additive solutions have a privileged status – they tend to come to mind quickly and easily." (Kwon, p. 16).

The poignant component of Adams et al. (2021) study for our discussion is that the addition of bricks can often look to be the focus, potentially privileging addition over subtraction. The importance of "subtraction" for my 8-year-old participant seemed paramount. They could have simply thrown the bricks around the room or tipped them out to make a noise, but there was something important in constructing *and* de-constructing. Both were important in helping them understand the interactivity of the parts of their creation. Sometimes, action is just for its joy. However, in the therapeutic context, we must remember that both construction and de-construction must be okay and safe, and both can have meaning within the therapeutic space.

Engage multiple senses

Sound

Building with LEGO® utilises the "clutch power" of the brick (Anthony, 2018; Skahill, 2020) (see Chapter 9 for more detail). Clutch power not only describes the connective strength of the design of the LEGO®

bricks as they are put together but also the sound that particular "click" they make when joining. There is tactile and auditory engagement when building. The hands hold, feel, and manipulate while the ears hear the connections. The cacophony can also bombard our ears as the hunt for just the right brick is undertaken, the crash of bricks whose clutch power has been weak or failed, or the vocalisation of the participant as the bricks accidentally or purposefully crash down.

Colour

One of the things I love about LEGO® is its colours. Kalbfleisch et al.'s (2013, pp. 55, 56) study, while not focussing on 3-D building, brings the dimension of colour into our discussions. The researchers report that using coloured objects vs black and white objects increases the retention of visual information in short-term memory and bridges conscious and non-conscious processing. Adding colour speeds up perceptual processing, "assists with object perception, . . . has a role in scene segmentation and visual memory, . . . decreases cognitive demand by alerting the brain to salient properties of the visual environment . . . and facilitates associative processing by boosting salience to support cognitive performance" – all essential aspects in the creation of metaphor and narrative.

Working in three dimensions (3-D)

LEGO® SERIOUS PLAY® (LSP), a keystone of STP, is a strategy that uses LEGO® to build a 3-D visual representation, assisting organisations to playfully improve their culture and performance (Wengel et al., 2021). The LSP 3-D-interview technique allows participants to get a more detailed view of the issue in a context that is not intimidating and externalised from the self – helping the participant visualise their understanding and share it with others. Programs like LEGO® Build-To-Express (Peabody, 2015) have assisted students in visualising and developing their knowledge of curriculum materials. The 3-D constructions help participants develop narratives and metaphors, facilitating their articulation of thoughts, making ideas explicit, and enhancing learning and understanding (James, 2013). Constructing with LEGO®, like making, crafting, drawing, and mapping, assists in externalising the mental models we create and helps make our understanding through metaphor constructed in the build explicitly. LEGO® bricklaying brings the creative process of 3-D "drawing" into everyone's reach; it is an easily accessible resource; "anyone can build with LEGO®." LEGO® is easy to use and shifts the making towards a more cohesive whole, allowing complex ideas to be more visible and at hand and helps the builder see things from different perspectives. The building enables us to touch, move around, and examine the spatial relationships – size, scale, depth, height and aspect. Like good artisans, LEGO® builders can create "a dialogue between concrete practices and thinking . . . establish[ing] a rhythm between problem-solving and problem-finding" (Sennett, 2009, p. 9).

A story I remembered from my biology teacher training highlights the impact of building 3-D models. The story centres around one of the most important discoveries of the 20th century: the 3-D model of DNA, developed from the work of Rosalind Franklin and made famous by Watson and Crick (Hernandez, 2019). Watson and Crick took Franklin's photographs (without her knowledge), provided the necessary measurements of DNA derived from Franklin's photo, and saw that the structure was a helix. Later, Watson obtained an internal university report written by Franklin and Click that concluded that the structure contained two strands – a double helix. However, they found the helix challenging to build. They had been working on the design for months with little success. Watson, now frustrated, took a leap of imagination and creativity:

> In desperation, I made some [models] out of cardboard. . . . I just used ordinary thin pieces of white covered smooth cardboard. . . . I made these six to nine member rings and then distinguished [the amino acids] and . . . I began moving them around, and I wanted an arrangement, you know, where I had a big and a small molecule . . . just switching around on the table [I saw] that adenine and thymine had formed a very nice base pair, and guanine and cytosine formed one identical in shape, and I thought you can build a double helix with adenine and thymine and guanine and cytosine base pairs. . . . The [base pairs] looked the same. And you could put one right on top of the other [three-dimensionally] . . . all fitting into this wonderful symmetry.
>
> (Watson, n.d.-a, n.d.-b)

To visualise their now-famous construction of the DNA double helix, Watson used manipulatives cut out of cardboard to create the 3-D model – *generating interactivity.*

Another innovative strategy that uses manipulatives and metaphors – this time, in coaching practice – is the "Metaphor Magic" process described by Lily Seto (Seto & Geithner, 2018). The approach has many of the hallmark features of Seriously Therapeutic Play (STP). Seto gives each participant a small box containing up to 25 randomly chosen "charms." During a session, the participant is asked to consider a question or situation they wish to explore and select an item(s) from the box representing that situation. The participant is then asked to describe the charm in context, developing a generative metaphor. The participant and coach then discuss the implications, learnings, and new perspectives offered by the generative metaphor the participant has articulated through an iterative process. Like the method used in STP, direct eye contact with the participant generally does not occur during this phase. The focus is on the object and the generative metaphor. The participant externalises their thinking and, to some degree, removes themselves from the issue(s). Again, like our STP process, manipulating the charm involves the participant somatically. Pick the charm up in their hand, physically manipulating it, and connecting it with other objects allows the participant to see things from a different perspective. The use of visual, auditory, or kinaesthetic channels engages more aspects of the brain. Seto asks the participant to check in with their "head, heart and gut," which facilitates "deeper learning."

Conclusion

A strategy I often use in therapy – and a perspective that warrants mention here – is the principle of KIS-MIF – "Keep it Simple, Make it Fun." Working with young children requires me to think at their level, not dumbing down because of their age but being clear and concise. Looking at the LEGO® builds of their interactions, which sometimes seem very complex to me, they often explain them in very straightforward terms. It is essential not to overanalyse and be in the moment with their descriptions and interpretations. I try to stay with "What can we take away from the construction that will make life easier for you?" Simply being in the moment with young people sometimes has little to do with what is happening outside our session and more to do with where they are in the moment.

One challenge when using manipulatives to pursue narrative and metaphor creation is that teachers and facilitators sometimes select an object from their stores. These may hold concrete or preconceived meanings; for example, the metaphor of the pizza slice as a fraction. A recent conversation with my daughter, a ski and snowboard instructor, reminded me of teaching my children to ski. We used "Pizza and Chips" to help them develop the skills of stopping (snow plough, pizza) and going (parallel, chips). She recently commented, "We don't use these metaphors anymore, as they encourage unhealthy eating!" We also need to be cautious about interpreting the participants meaning behind any manipulative (see Figure 0.1 in the introduction chapter as an example).

It is also essential to consider that a manipulative may contain specific or multiple meanings. Willingham (2017, pp. 29, 30) comments that working memory can be overwhelmed when objects have multiple meanings. "Perceptually rich objects draw attention to themselves, which can be" useful if the richness relates to the task. However, they are more useful if the objects are "abstract symbols." In therapy, this richness needs to be attributed by the participant to the narrative and metaphors. We believe LEGO® bricks meet the criteria as many "bricks" are abstract symbols having no preconceived meaning. A brick is a brick; it can be a rich object whose purpose arises from the representation that the participant employs.

The hand-mind connection has a very significant history in the development of the physiological structures of the brain, including the speech centres and the five-finger grip (opposable thumb), which coevolved. "The hand is not simply an evolutionary curiosity, . . . but an important part of the developing powers of human cognition." (Bürgi et al., 2005, p. 80) Through serious play, we believe we can assist participants to deeply explore their worldview with their hands and through metaphor. Chapter 2 further explores the research underpinning our understanding of brain development. We further discuss the DMN and TPN and their importance in supporting our contention that STP provides an excellent avenue for participants to develop their understanding of their world and see things afresh.

References

Adams, G. S., Converse, B. A., Hales, A. H., & Klotz, L. E. (2021). People systematically overlook subtractive changes. *Nature, 592*(7853), Article 7853. https://doi.org/10.1038/s41586-021-03380-y

Anthony, W. (2018). The LEGO story. *Scandinavian Review*, 17–33.

Australian Curriculum, Assessment and Reporting Authority (ACARA). (2022). *Australian curriculum key ideas.* www.australiancurriculum.edu.au/f-10-curriculum/mathematics/key-ideas/

Avdi, E., & Seikkula, J. (2019). Studying the process of psychoanalytic psychotherapy: Discursive and embodied aspects. *British Journal of Psychotherapy, 35*(2), 217–232. https://doi.org/10.1111/bjp.12444

Bambini, V., Gentili, C., Ricciardi, E., Bertinetto, P. M., & Pietrini, P. (2011). Decomposing metaphor processing at the cognitive and neural level through functional magnetic resonance imaging. *Brain Research Bulletin, 86*(3–4), 203–216. https://doi.org/10.1016/j.brainresbull.2011.07.015

Banaji, M. R. R., & Greenwald, A. G. (2016). *Blindspot: Hidden biases of good people* (Reprint ed.). Random House Publishing Group.

Barton, G., & James, A. (2017). Threshold concepts, LEGO® SERIOUS PLAY® and whole systems thinking: Towards a combined methodology. *Practice and Evidence of Scholarship of Teaching and Learning in Higher Education Special Issue: Threshold Concepts and Conceptual Difficulty, 12*(2), 23.

Beaty, R. E., Benedek, M., Wilkins, R. W., Jauk, E., Fink, A., Silvia, P. J., Hodges, D. A., Koschutnig, K., & Neubauer, A. C. (2014). Creativity and the default network: A functional connectivity analysis of the creative brain at rest. *Neuropsychologia, 64*, 92–98. https://doi.org/10.1016/j.neuropsychologia.2014.09.019

Bürgi, P. T., Jacobs, C. D., & Roos, J. (2005). From metaphor to practice: In the crafting of strategy. *Journal of Management Inquiry, 14*(1), 78–94. https://doi.org/10.1177/1056492604270802

Chabris, C., & Simons, D. (2011). *The invisible gorilla: How our intuitions deceive us* (Reprint ed.). Harmony. www.theinvisiblegorilla.com/videos.html

Christoff, K., Irving, Z. C., Fox, K. C. R., Spreng, R. N., & Andrews-Hanna, J. R. (2016). Mind-wandering as spontaneous thought: A dynamic framework. *Nature Reviews Neuroscience, 17*(11), 718–731. https://doi.org/10.1038/nrn.2016.113

Cieri, F., & Esposito, R. (2019). Psychoanalysis and neuroscience: The bridge between mind and brain. *Frontiers in Psychology, 10*. www.frontiersin.org/article/10.3389/fpsyg.2019.01983

Dekker, S., Lee, N., Howard-Jones, P., & Jolles, J. (2012). Neuromyths in education: Prevalence and predictors of misconceptions among teachers. *Frontiers in Psychology, 3*. www.frontiersin.org/article/10.3389/fpsyg.2012.00429

Dunn, M. (2021). Research: Is a picture worth 1,000 words or 60,000 words in marketing? *Email Audience.* www.emailaudience.com/research-picture-worth-1000-words-marketing/

Egan, G., & Reese, R. J. (2018). *The skilled helper: A problem-management and opportunity-development approach to helping.* Cengage Learning.

Eliot, L. (2019). Bad science and the unisex brain. *Nature, 566*(7745), 453–454. https://doi.org/10.1038/d41586-019-00677-x

Eliot, L., Ahmed, A., Khan, H., & Patel, J. (2021). Dump the "dimorphism": Comprehensive synthesis of human brain studies reveals few male-female differences beyond size. *Neuroscience & Biobehavioral Reviews, 125,* 667–697. https://doi.org/10.1016/j.neubiorev.2021.02.026

Friston, K. (2016). *Free energy principle.* Serious Science. http://serious-science.org/free-energy-principle-7602

Gauntlett, D. (2018). *Making is connecting: The social power of creativity, from craft and knitting to digital everything.* John Wiley & Sons.

Hagen, S. (2012). The mind's eye. *Rochester Review, 74*(4). www.rochester.edu/pr/Review/V74N4/0402_brainscience.html

Hernandez, V. (2019). Photograph 51, by Rosalind Franklin (1952). *Embryo Project Encyclopedia, 4.*

Hipólito, I., Ramstead, M. J. D., Convertino, L., Bhat, A., Friston, K., & Parr, T. (2021). Markov blankets in the brain. *Neuroscience and Biobehavioral Reviews, 125,* 88–97. https://doi.org/10.1016/j.neubiorev.2021.02.003

Holmes, J., & Nolte, T. (2019). "Surprise" and the Bayesian brain: Implications for psychotherapy theory and practice. *Frontiers in Psychology, 10,* 592. https://doi.org/10.3389/fpsyg.2019.00592

Huff, A. S., & Jenkins, M. (2002). *Mapping strategic knowledge.* SAGE Publications.

Isomura, T., Shimazaki, H., & Friston, K. J. (2022). Canonical neural networks perform active inference. *Communications Biology, 5*(1), 55. https://doi.org/10.1038/s42003-021-02994-2

James, A. R. (2013). LEGO® SERIOUS PLAY®: A three-dimensional approach to learning development. *Journal of Learning Development in Higher Education, 6.* https://doi.org/10.47408/jldhe.v0i6.208

Jenkins, A. C. (2019). Rethinking cognitive load: A default-mode network perspective. *Trends in Cognitive Sciences, 23*(7), 531–533. https://doi.org/10.1016/j.tics.2019.04.008

Kalbfleisch, L., DeBettencourt, M., Kopperman, R., Banasiak, M., Roberts, J., & Halavi, M. (2013). Environmental influences on neural systems of relational complexity. *Frontiers in Psychology, 4.* www.frontiersin.org/article/10.3389/fpsyg.2013.00631

Kristiansen, P., & Rasmussen, R. (2014). *Building a better business using the LEGO® SERIOUS PLAY® method.* John Wiley & Sons.

Kuhn, S. (2022). *Transforming learning through tangible instruction* (0 ed.). Routledge. https://doi.org/10.4324/9781003129073

Kwon, D. (2021). Our brain typically overlooks this brilliant problem-solving strategy. *Scientific American Mind, 32*(4), 14–16.

Laber-Warren, E. (2022). Aha! Moments pop up from below the level of conscious awareness. *Scientific American, 33*(3), 6–7.

Lampert, M. (1988). What can research on teacher education tell us about improving quality in mathematics education? *Teaching and Teacher Education, 4*(2), 157–170. https://doi.org/10.1016/0742-051X(88)90015-7

Lovitt, C., & Lowe, I. (1984). *RIME lesson pack: Reality in mathematics education teacher development project*. Research and Development Curriculum Branch, Education Department of Victoria.

Manassi, M., & Whitney, D. (2022). Illusion of visual stability through active perceptual serial dependence. *Science Advances, 8*(2), eabk2480. https://doi.org/10.1126/sciadv.abk2480

Mercê, C., Branco, M., Catela, D., Lopes, F., & Cordovil, R. (2022). Learning to cycle: From training wheels to balance bike. *International Journal of Environmental Research and Public Health, 19*(3), 1814. https://doi.org/10.3390/ijerph19031814

Nielsen, J. A., Zielinski, B. A., Ferguson, M. A., Lainhart, J. E., & Anderson, J. S. (2013). An evaluation of the left-brain vs. right-brain hypothesis with resting state functional connectivity magnetic resonance imaging. *PLoS One, 8*(8), e71275. https://doi.org/10.1371/journal.pone.0071275

OECD. (n.d.-a). *Neuromyth 3 – OECD*. Retrieved April 11, 2022, from www.oecd.org/education/ceri/neuromyth3.htm

OECD. (n.d.-b). *Neuromyth 6 – OECD*. Centre for Educational Research and Innovation (CERI). Retrieved April 11, 2022, from www.oecd.org/education/ceri/neuromyth6.htm

Paul, A. M. (2021). *The extended mind: The power of thinking outside the brain*. Houghton Mifflin Harcourt.

Peabody, M. A. (2015). Building with purpose: Using LEGO® SERIOUS PLAY® in play therapy supervision. *International Journal of Play Therapy, 24*(1), 30–40. https://doi.org/10.1037/a0038607

Quillin, K., & Thomas, S. (2015). Drawing-to-learn: A framework for using drawings to promote model-based reasoning in biology. *CBE – Life Sciences Education, 14*(1), es2. https://doi.org/10.1187/cbe.14-08-0128

Rapp, A. M., Mutschler, D. E., & Erb, M. (2012). Where in the brain is nonliteral language? A coordinate-based meta-analysis of functional magnetic resonance imaging studies. *NeuroImage, 63*(1), 600–610. https://doi.org/10.1016/j.neuroimage.2012.06.022

Salazar Kämpf, M., Nestler, S., Hansmeier, J., Glombiewski, J., & Exner, C. (2021). Mimicry in psychotherapy – an actor partner model of therapists' and patients' non-verbal behavior and its effects on the working alliance. *Psychotherapy Research, 31*(6), 752–764. https://doi.org/10.1080/10503307.2020.1849849

Schmidgall, S. P., Scheiter, K., & Eitel, A. (2020). Can we further improve tablet-based drawing to enhance learning? An empirical test of two types of support. *Instructional Science, 48*(4), 453–474. https://doi.org/10.1007/s11251-020-09513-6

Schön, D. A. (1993). Generative metaphor: A perspective on problem-setting in social policy. In A. Ortony (Ed.), *Metaphor and thought* (2nd ed., pp. 137–163). Cambridge University Press. https://doi.org/10.1017/CBO9781139173865.011

Sennett, R. (2009). *The Craftsman*. Penguin UK.

Seto, L., & Geithner, T. (2018). Metaphor magic in coaching and coaching supervision. *International Journal of Evidence Based Coaching and Mentoring, 16*(2), 99–111. https://doi.org/10.24384/000562

Skahill, S. (2020). Surprising discovery about Godtfred Kirk Christiansen revealed on his 100th birthday. *LEGO Ambassador Network.* https://lan.lego.com/news/overview/surprising-discovery-about-godtfred-kirk-christiansen-revealed-on-his-100th-birthday-r265/

Smallwood, J., Gorgolewski, K. J., Golchert, J., Ruby, F. J. M., Engen, H., Baird, B., Vinski, M. T., Schooler, J. W., & Margulies, D. S. (2013). The default modes of reading: Modulation of posterior cingulate and medial prefrontal cortex connectivity associated with comprehension and task focus while reading. *Frontiers in Human Neuroscience, 7*, 734. https://doi.org/10.3389/fnhum.2013.00734

Stickley, T. (2011). From SOLER to SURETY for effective non-verbal communication. *Nurse Education in Practice, 11*(6), 395–398. https://doi.org/10.1016/j.nepr.2011.03.021

Stuyck, H., Cleeremans, A., & Van den Bussche, E. (2022). Aha! under pressure: The Aha! experience is not constrained by cognitive load. *Cognition, 219*, 104946. https://doi.org/10.1016/j.cognition.2021.104946

Trafton, A. (2014). In the blink of an eye. *MIT News.* https://news.mit.edu/2014/in-the-blink-of-an-eye-0116

van Eijk, L., Zhu, D., Couvy-Duchesne, B., Strike, L. T., Lee, A. J., Hansell, N. K., Thompson, P. M., de Zubicaray, G. I., McMahon, K. L., Wright, M. J., & Zietsch, B. P. (2021). Are sex differences in human brain structure associated with sex differences in behavior? *Psychological Science, 32*(8), 1183–1197. https://doi.org/10.1177/0956797621996664

Watson, J. (Director). (n.d.-a). *Discovering the double helix structure, James Watson.* Retrieved October 24, 2021, from https://dnalc.cshl.edu/view/15452-Discovering-the-double-helix-structure-James-Watson.html

Watson, J. (Director). (n.d.-b). *Discovering the double helix structure of DNA, James Watson, video with 3D animation and narration: CSHL DNA Learning Center.* Retrieved October 24, 2021, from https://dnalc.cshl.edu/view/15492-Discovering-the-double-helix-structure-of-DNA-James-Watson-video-with-3D-animation-and-narration.html

Wengel, Y., McIntosh, A., & Cockburn-Wootten, C. (2021). A critical consideration of LEGO® SERIOUS PLAY® methodology for tourism studies. *Tourism Geographies, 23*(1–2), 162–184. https://doi.org/10.1080/14616688.2019.1611910

Willingham, D. T. (2017, Fall). Ask the cognitive scientist: Do manipulatives help students learn? *American Educator, 7.*

CHAPTER 2
THE NEUROSCIENCE OF PLAY

Alec Hamilton

A foundation underpinning of Seriously Therapeutic Play with LEGO® (STP) is that we can all play to examine our reality via our hands; specifically, with LEGO® bricks; we can build our perception, thoughts, emotions, and problems and explore ourselves. This form of play allows us to connect with ourselves and others. We can step away somewhat from the seriousness of the issues we face and create something that can inform us about ourselves. We believe building three-dimensional models as a metaphor is linked with expressing imagination, problem-solving, innovative thinking, testing ideas, and exploring identity. We explored these ideas in depth in Chapter 1. It is, perhaps, not by chance that we are writing this book during the COVID-19 pandemic when the connections with ourselves and with each other have been strained. This chapter explores our current understanding of neuroscience and how it informs our understanding of our connections with ourselves and each other. We will link this scientific understanding of the neural networks to play and further introduce the reader to how using LEGO® in therapy to build, construct, and think with our hands has therapeutic value, allowing us to understand our world afresh.

DOI: 10.4324/9781003260424-3

The neuroscience of human connection

This chapter is early in the book because we thought we needed to start with our current understanding of how the brain works; we believe we know a fair bit about the mechanism operating in the brain; however, this knowledge is in the nascence stages. For example, when I started studying psychology some 30 years ago, I was taught that adults' brains were fixed and that the idea of neuroplasticity was never mentioned. I was surprised to learn, some years later, that the notion of neuroplasticity first appeared in the literature at the beginning of the 20th century (Fuchs & Flügge, 2014), long before I was in undergraduate school, and debate around a fixed or flexible brain structure continued for many years. Sadly, my professors must have been on the side of a fixed view of the brain. Consequently, early 1990s novice psychologists like me saw our clients' cognitive abilities as fixed – for life. Being open to different understandings of the brain and its workings is as essential today as it was then. We mention this here to highlight that many of the ideas presented in the pages that follow are based on the dominant and current science – the identifiable, best evidence. However, the field is dynamic and changing rapidly. It is essential to recognise that we are all making connections based on what we see and currently understand in neuroscience and from our respective therapeutic experiences.

How the brain grows: neurogenesis, neuroplasticity and neuro-pruning

Three key processes occur within the brain that assists individuals in understanding and managing their world: neurogenesis, neuroplasticity, and neuro-pruning. Neurogenesis is the brain's ability to grow new neural pathways and networks. Neuroplasticity refers to the brain's ability to reform connections and rewire the already-developed neural pathways and networks (Maharjan et al., 2020). Building neural pathways and networks through neurogenesis and neuroplasticity is captured in the phrase "fire together, wire together" – an abridged version of Hebb's theory (1949). When neurons actively work together, the developed pathways become stronger and more efficient, building more robust connections – i.e., we learn. Neuro-pruning involves a reduction in the synaptic connection and works parallel with the other two processes; as one pathway builds, others diminish and are eventually pruned away. Neurogenesis and neuroplasticity start early in pregnancy and continue into adulthood (Queensland Brain Institute, 2016). Neuro-pruning starts a little later. Jeff Lichtman (Sakai, 2020, p. 16096), a neuroscientist at Harvard University, is reported to have said,

> you start wired up for every possible contingency, . . . over time, a large percentage of those wires are permanently disconnected, . . . and you're left with a narrower nervous system, . . . tuned exactly to the world you found yourself in.

From a therapeutic perspective, this is the self that arrives in therapy. This self has developed a neurological system tuned explicitly for and by the experiences and environment in which it has lived. It is this nervous system, with its "connectopathies" – aberrant neural connections – that we are trying to help clients modify and adapt to the world in which they wish to live.

The connection between the structure and the function of the brain – "structure-function coupling" (wiring and firing) – is highlighted in a study by Baum et al. (2020) and Social Brain Theory (Dunbar & Shultz, 2017). Baum et al. examined the neuroimaging data of 727 young people aged 8 to 23. They observed "that functional communication was directly supported by local white-matter pathways" (p. 775) – i.e., "architecture" was linked to "activity"; *wiring was connected to firing*. Furthermore, "age-related increases in coupling were disproportionately enriched within the default mode network" (DMN), with strong coupling shown within parts of the DMN. The DMN and Social Brain Theory are discussed in more detail later.

Many facilitators are probably not overly concerned with the specifics of what is happening structurally in the client's brain. Instead, they focus on how we might help our clients develop new ways of being. However, it is important to know that the brain needs to undo some connections while re-building and building other pathways. Any shift backwards and forwards in behaviour and thinking represents an outward representation of what is happening structurally in the brain. The following section looks at our understanding of the neural pathways developed in childhood and modified and pruned as we grow, emphasising the importance of play.

Important brain networks

The challenge for many facilitators is to link research, theory, and practice. Here, the challenge is connecting the brain's structure to the functional descriptions made earlier about the social brain. We believe two specific neural pathways, or brain networks – The Default Mode Network and the Task Positive Network – make this connection, and they will be discussed in the following section. Their importance for understanding LEGO® play in therapy will emerge.

Default Mode Network

The Default Mode Network (DMN) was first described as a "resting state" (Raichle, 2015; Raichle et al., 2001) because it was observed when a person was resting quietly with their eyes closed. The DMN involves, in the main, the posterior cingulate cortex (PCC), medial prefrontal cortex (MPFC) (Smallwood, Bernhardt, et al., 2021), and has also been described as the "social brain" (Moran et al., 2013, p. 1). It has also been suggested that the DMN involves parts of the limbic circuitry (Li et al., 2014).

The DMN assists us in having stimulus-independent, conscious experiences, helping us process semantic and conceptual information, time travel (past and future), develop conceptual judgements about our world, and generate predictions based on our memories. The DMN is involved in constructing our internal worldview, or "mental maps." These maps are acquired from the long-term memories we have created about ourselves, others, and the world around us and are associated with social cognition (Hughes et al., 2019; Li et al., 2014; Mars et al., 2012). Social cognition is a complex system and involves "self-relevant affective" decision-making (Li et al., p. 5), self-understanding, social behaviour, empathy, emotional perception and responses, visual self-recognition, self-control, and ethical decision-making. Social cognition involves obtaining, retrieving, and processing information about ourselves and our relationships but also assists in helping us to understand the mental states of others (Mars et al., 2012, p. 3). The ability to understand others, their emotions, and mental and psychological states and predict another's behaviour is described as the "Theory of Mind" (ToM). ToM can be viewed as a subset of social cognition and is a vital "skill" required for social interaction. DMN plays a crucial role in synthesising and integrating information from our social world (Tylén et al., 2015), assisting personal perspectives to be adapted towards developing models of others' social behaviour – ToM. These internal models are continuously updated and guide our attention. The DMN attempts to predict or foretell what will develop in our environment based on these models and our understanding of others by cycling between "monitoring and correcting" based on errors or success in its predictions (Smallwood, Bernhardt, et al., 2021, p. 510).

The DMN also plays a broader role than just social cognition and is involved in developing positive emotions, creativity, openness to new ideas, emotional self-awareness and insightful problem-solving (Boyatzis et al., 2014, 2015). It is goal oriented and involved in "constructive processes of multi-episode integration, imagining the future and mental scene construction . . . *plot formation*" (Tylén et al., 2015, p. 107, emphasis in original). The MFPC assists the DMN to shift between externally focussed awareness of others and internally focussed processes – awareness of self. The MFPC works as a conduit, taking sensory information and acting as the "desktop," consciously guiding our in-the-moment thoughts (Moran et al., 2013). This ability to shift attention from internal to external assists in distinguishing between self and other and facilitates recognising another's mental state and inferring their emotionality. The DMN, through the MFPC, has a strong connection with the amygdala, which helps regulate mental and socioemotional states and facilitates our understanding of the emotional connections during social interactions. Play with self and others allows us to shift between external and internal, assisting us to understand the world and act out the stories we develop. Play helps us experience emotions within a relatively safe context and acts as a functional mechanism for the MFPC. We believe that the STP facilitates this external-internal interplay via the development of block metaphors that assist us in representing our internal conscious and unconscious imaginings externally.

Questions have been raised from a developmental standpoint about DMN in children. Both Chaddock-Heyman et al. (2018) and Camacho et al. (2020) report differences in the DMN of adults and children. Chaddock-Heyman et al. found that connectivity between the PCC and MPFC is less mature in children (7- to 9-year-olds). Those children with higher scholastic achievement showed greater connectivity than their less-scholastic peers, suggesting they were illustrating a shift towards a more adult DMN. Camacho et al. indicate that neural activity is unfolding much faster in young children due to neural plasticity. Therefore, one would expect children to have much greater spontaneous neural activity

driving structural and functional changes during this time of foundational brain development. From this perspective, we would expect a
child's neural activity to be more akin to finding interest in a random jigsaw puzzle piece as they develop the pathways to understand the concept
of the jigsaw as a whole. We see this in babies' apparent spontaneous foot
and hand finding and the joy of placing these in the mouth, at first by
chance, then through planned action, as the neural pathway of deliberate
behaviour develops. Practitioners working in early childhood learning
centres are well aware of similar behaviour in the spontaneous singing
and chatting of 4- to 8-year-olds and recognise how these behaviours are
often associated with play rather than a cognitive task.

Weaker connections within the DMN have been linked to aging and
declines in one's theory of mind abilities and may also be related to
issues with self-referential thinking (Hughes et al., 2019). Altered connections or more time within the DMN have been reported in people
with ADHD, Alzheimer's, depression, autism, and schizophrenia (Atzil
et al., 2018; Raichle, 2010; Smallwood et al., 2013).

Task Positive Network

The second brain network, the Task Positive Network (TPN), comprises
various areas of the brain, including the Prefrontal Cortex (PFC), and
is active during cognitive tasks that require attention and external focus,
which are essential for problem-solving, working memory, decision-making, controlling actions in the external world (Boyatzis et al., 2015), and
creativity (Sun et al., 2019). There is some contention within neuroscience about the specific structures included in the TPN, what to name the
network, and if this is a network in itself or a combination of networks
(see Witt et al., 2021). The choice made here has arisen from a particle
perspective; viewing the TPN as a single network has been helpful in my
therapeutic work. Using the label "TPN" serves a purpose, as it helps
explain the actions a participant may need to undertake to engage their
full undivided attention.

I first became aware of the DMN and TPN when they were initially
referred to as "task-positive" and "task-negative." As the research developed, the label "DMN" took over from "task-negative," as it more precisely describes the network's actions. The research on the TPN remains
unclear, and there are concerns with the label. Deming (2021) and Witt
et al. (2021) indicate that there is a diversity of names being used to

describe what we have chosen to name the TPN: "central executive network (CEN), cognitive control network (CCN), dorsal attention network (DAN), executive control network (ECN), executive network (EN), frontoparietal network (FPN), frontoparietal control network (FPCN), working memory network (WMN), and ventral attention network (VAN)" (Witt et al., p. 5).

Furthermore, Witt et al. (2021) indicate that the ECN, DAN, and FPN, are separate networks; however, authors use various labels to describe visually similar brain areas. The task of resolving these issues is outside our scope. Therefore, our decision on the name TPN is once again a practical one. TPN captures the understanding reported by Deming (2021) that the TPN "network" represents the interaction of the Frontoparietal Network (FPN) and the Salience Network (SN). In the discussions that follow, when we refer to the TPN, we reference both the FPN and SN. However, we think it is important to pause and discuss the relevance of the FPN and SN as separate networks to help understand the process occurring within the brain.

Frontoparietal Network

The Frontoparietal Network (FPN) involves the dorsolateral prefrontal cortex (dPFC) and posterior parietal cortex (pPC). It is engaged in externally focussed cognitively demanding tasks that require sustained attention, complex problem-solving, and manipulating working memory. Activity in the FPN (and the SN) is diminished when there is an increase in activity in the DMN and vice versa.

Salience Network

The Salience Network (SN) includes the ventrolateral prefrontal cortex (vlPFC), the fronto-insular cortex (FIC), and the anterior cingulate cortex (ACC). It is engaged when cognitively demanding tasks that require detection and attention to salient (noticeable) clues and goal-seeking behaviour. The network receives external inputs (visual, kinaesthetic, and auditory) for their integration. The ACC "plays a key role in affective evaluation, conflict monitoring and detection, response selection, and attentional control" (Cieri & Esposito, 2019, p. 7). Deming (2021) suggests that the SN assists in the switch between the DMN and FPN.

Furthermore, the SN has a diminished role in those who are experiencing psychopathology (Deming, 2021). Deming found that errors in sensing the external environment (i.e., issues with the SN) could reduce communication between the ACC and the FPN. These errors reduce the excitatory response of the FPN and the inhibitory response of the DMN. When the SN does not notice, the FPN fails to get the message to respond and the DMN fails to get the message to decrease its involvement. Interestingly, Krönke et al. (2020), in their study of participants without known psychopathology, found that SN regulation of interchanged between the DMN and the FPN is an integral part of real-life self-control. Errors in the SN also fit with reports that reduced cognitive control is observed in depression, OCD, ADHD, and anxiety.

The relationship between DMN and TPN

In simple terms, the DMN has an antagonistic relationship with the TPN. I describe the relationship between the TPN and DMN to younger clients: "when one is off, the other is on." A more complex explanation suggests a dynamic process of shifting between two poles – DMN and TPN (Smallwood, Turnbull, et al., 2021; Spreng, 2012). Rather than being purely antagonistic, the two networks appear to work together. They can switch like the clutch and accelerator of a car, manoeuvring between the networks as the needs of the external or internal worlds take priority. The graded manoeuvring between the DMN and TPN appears to be essential for managing our environment and emphasises SN's role. Functionally, the process can be described as the TPN observing and acting on the environment (SN notices, and the FPN responds). The DMN is then involved in linking the external stimuli from the TPN with what is already known and predicts what might happen in the future. The DMN and TPN work together to create "more integrated forms of cognition" and contribute to "spontaneous thoughts" and "spontaneous self-generated states" and connect "detailed, or immersive experiences," helping establish a sense of in-the-moment "presence" (Smallwood, Turnbull, et al., pp. 8, 12).

DMN appears to be required to understand social processes or when information stored in memory might contribute to ongoing thoughts and help manage tasks within the external world (Smallwood, Turnbull, et al., 2021). The DMN assigns value to the internal concept created by an external stimulus and builds on the idea from an egocentric perspective. Smallwood et al. report that the DMN might be involved in "mental time travel," tapping into episodic and semantic memory, particularly when the TPN requires information to complete external tasks.

Kucyi et al. (2016) propose that, while spontaneous DMN activity reflects internal mental processes, the activity is only partially connected to mind wandering and may be influenced by internal/external attention fluctuations. Baum et al. (2020) proposed that the strong structural-functional coupling with the DMN may reduce "competitive interference" from the TPN, "allowing for the suppression of internally generated thoughts while maintaining and manipulating information in working memory" (p. 775). Takeuchi et al. (2013, p. 325) speculate that individuals with higher interpersonal emotional intelligence may show increased regulation of DMN through parts of TPN. They reported that higher trait emotional intelligence was associated with greater functional connectivity in critical areas of the DMN and social cognition. Furthermore, the brain's ability to switch between DMN (creative internal thinking, "novel metaphor production, goal-directed memory retrieval"), suppress old thoughts ("prepotent-response inhibition") and TPN (process information from the outside world) are paramount in creativity (Beaty et al., 2019; Rubinstein & Lahad, 2022, p. 2; Sun et al., 2019)

The link between DMN, TPN, and play

The brain in play

Liu et al. (2017, p. 3; see also Zosh et al., 2018) reviewed the neuroscience and biological literature on learning and play. They outline five characteristics of playful learning:

- Joy is integral to brain networks responsible for learning.
- Meaningful experiences introduce novel stimuli linking the known with the unknown; internal with external.
- Active engagement develops cognitive control attention and enhances memory.
- Iteration increases the ability to develop alternative perspectives, flexible thinking, and creativity.
- Social interaction activates brain networks related to detecting the mental states of others – Theory of Mind (ToM).

Joy

Liu et al. (2017) report that brain networks, including the PFC, ACC, and PCC, respond adaptively to joyful play experiences. Joy and other positive emotions are associated with higher levels of neurotransmitters like dopamine. Experiences of joy and other emotions reveal changes in the DMN, the ACC, and the amygdala (aspects of the SN) (Li et al., 2014). Increases in dopamine enhance working memory, attention, mental shifting, creativity, and improved self-regulation – all requirements and characteristic of DMN/TPN interaction. These chemical and brain activations highlight the likelihood that during play, the brain engages in emotional responses and moves from self-referential to externally focussed and back again.

Meaningful activities

The importance of meaningful activities for learning is well supported by research on motivation and development. Liu et al. (2017) indicate that meaningful play allows for the development of new knowledge and the confirmation or modification of prior learning. Luu et al. (2007) suggest that two circuits identified in animal studies are associated with learning. "Rapid learning" involves several cortical areas, including the ACC and amygdala, and assists attention and evaluation for inconsistencies with prior knowledge or foretelling of an outcome. The "late-stage" system is centred on the PCC and fits the new learning into prior learning. Both systems act like the network model described above and engage cortical areas associated with the DMN and TPN.

Active engagement

To actively engage in something, one must be engrossed, attentive, focussed, and responsive. The ability to attend to something outside oneself and be engaged in a task requires deep concentration. Ruckli (2016) tentatively proposes that deep engagement – a flow state – may quieten the DMN. The flow state (Csikszentmihalyi, 2008) is, perhaps, the ultimate state of engagement (see Chapter 4 for a more details discussion of flow). To be in flow, a task must be challenging, *and* the individual must have the skill and experience to undertake the task. Flow states can only occur when there is "just the right balance" of skill and challenge. Wright et al. (2014) describe flow within the context of Reversal Theory, which can provide a structure/function link with the DMN and TPN.

Reversal Theory (Apter, 1997) proposes several different but universal ways of experiencing the world. These "experiential" states occur in pairs of opposites, with only one of the pairs in operation at a time. We switch, or "reverse," between the two states. Apter reported that there are four pairs of states. The pair most relevant to our discussion is the telic/paratelic states. The telic state is goal orientated and is a "serious-minded state" where we are focussed and engaged in a meaningful, important activity "beyond itself." The paratelic state is a "playful" activity that is enjoyable in itself. Apter notes that one can switch between the states within one activity, switching from playful to serious and back again.

> In the telic state, one becomes anxious as threatening or demanding events raise arousal levels but is pleasantly relaxed when a task is completed. In the paratelic state, one becomes pleasantly excited as one becomes more emotionally involved and aroused but bored if there is a lack of stimulation.
>
> (para. 19)

In a study by Wright et al. (2014), flow experiences were linked with paratelic and telic states. Paratelic flow occurred when people experienced joy within the context of high arousal levels, and as their skill improved, their level of enjoyment increased. Wright et al. suggest this may be due to the participants shifting out of their worries and concerns, consistent with a shift from DMN to TPN. In contrast, telic flow resulted from self-focussed activities and generally centred on attempting to master something themselves. One participant commented that state helped them relax, consistent with shifting from task-positive to self-focussed.

Play allows us to shift from a telic, or serious, state to a paratelic, or playful, state of mind, helping us focus on the activity at hand and enjoy its challenges. Play is less goal focussed and more exploratory and enjoyment focussed. The paratelic state is necessary for strategy work (our notion of "serious play") in that it permits the exploration of ideas for a future that does not yet exist, possibly relying on the DMN. The back and forward movement from paratelic to telic fits with the observations made by clients when working with STP.

> I start by thinking about what I'm doing. I think I'm in control of it. I'm being intentional. Then I gradually changed my mind and started changing things and reorganising them. I start to add items without really thinking about them, and it starts to develop and becomes – Then, when I begin to narrate, I start to see things I did not notice, and that is when I know I have not consciously con-

trolled it. The model is more than I was consciously controlling. The skilled questioning during the narrative phase helps me discover what I am looking at and allows me to see things differently.

Iterative

Humans actively engage in the process of watching the world, building stories or maps about it, using what they know to explore and refine their knowledge and then predicting and creating more refined maps of the world. This iterative process is seen when young children focus on objects that "violate" what they know (Zosh et al., 2018). Play "inspires iteration" (p. 7) and allows children to explore and build their knowledge, particularly when play involves social interaction. When play increases in complexity and people have the necessary skills, they like the activity more and are prepared to spend more time on the activity. Children's "guided play," which involves exploration within boundaries, as opposed to structured, adult-led play, also facilitates this iterative process. Building stories and maps require the individual to mentally represent the events, write and store memories, and develop a perspective which in turn sets us up to make predictions and foretell the future. Paying attention to a task, taking in external information, processing, storing it, and making it one's own matches the DMN/TPN process outlined earlier.

Social interaction

Atzil et al. (2018) suggest that core social knowledge develops from learning about social interactions within self and with others. Development of our social selves begins as rudimentary schemas, building to more complex "conceptual systems." A vital aspect of developing this conceptual system is the internal-external back and forward transfer of information. We would expect a baby's ability to predict the world would be limited. Then, as the child develops, their "internal predictive systems" and "external explorative systems" would improve. This has been observed in the studies reported above (Liu et al., 2017; Luu et al., 2007) and is consistent with the social brain theory discussed previously.

Atzil et al.'s (2018) comments match the results reported by Camacho et al. (2020), who indicate that the task-positive and task-negative responses in children (associated with the TPN and DMN in adults) shift across the first year of life and into the toddler years. The resting state in children appears to be different to that of adults. Parts of the DMN and the FPN are more strongly connected in children and distinctly separate in adults, while other connections within the DMN network strengthen during adolescence (Barber et al., 2013). The resting state is consistent with "cognitively waiting" in young children. The child "rests," waiting for the next meaningful input or feedback on predictions. In the child, this brain activity is more affiliated with task-positive rather than the prediction/evaluation process of the DMN seen in older children and adults. The inhibitory response is also insufficiently developed in young children up to 8 years old (Camacho et al.), resulting in more spontaneous behaviour actively driving neurological development. As children develop, around 10 years of age, they start to develop the cognitive flexibility and the prefrontal cortex development and DMN/TPN dynamic we see in adults.

The shifting TPN/DMN we observe in childhood parallels Alison Gopnik's (Gopnik, 2011a) work describing the contrast between how babies and young children attend to their outside world and how adults attend: "Children explore, adults exploit." (Gopnik, 2017) She proposes that, for adults, one form of consciousness or focus looks like a "spotlight"; "we decide that something's relevant or important, we should pay attention to it. Our consciousness of that thing that we're attending to becomes extremely bright and vivid, and everything else sort of goes dark" (Gopnik, 2011b, sec. 15:25). The PFC (DMN) sends a signal via the SN, "narrowing" the brain's focus and attention, resulting in more goal or task focus (TPN). In contrast, Gopnik proposes that babies and young children struggle with spotlight focus and, instead, use "lantern" focusing. They take on a broader view of their surroundings "they're flooded with these neurotransmitters that are really good at inducing learning and plasticity, and the inhibitory parts [probably the SN] have not come on yet." Gopnik's description parallels Camacho et al.'s (2020) comments earlier, where young children "cognitively wait" and broadly focus on their world, ready to take in as much as possible.

Gopnik (2021) also highlights the influence of attention when we experience awe or are fully engrossed in a movie or book, and we "lose ourselves" and our sense of time when we are in flow. Awe experiences, she suggests, are like lantern consciousness with neither the DMN nor the full TPN activated. This is supported by Van Elk et al. (2019), who report that the FPN network is strongly activated during awe-inspiring videos, compared to positive and neutral videos. The implications they draw is that the self-referential aspect of a task-positive activity has decreased or stopped – the self is lost – which we suggest is consistent with a decrease in the SN's switching process and disconnection of the DMN, and this "looks more like the child's brain" (Gopnik, 2021, sec. 15:27). Adults can also achieve the lantern consciousness of a child during play. Play is "another way of having this explore state of being in the world . . . hard-headed [AI] engineers . . . increasingly realize that play is something that's going to actually be able to get you systems that do better in going through the world" (sec. 23.33).

Why do you need to know all this neuro-psych stuff?

As facilitators, we like to know why something operates in the way it does. Often, we do not need to know everything; we need enough to understand the rationale and the research evidence behind our interventions. In this chapter, we have presented, we believe, a convincing argument for how the DMN-TPN dynamic represents an excellent model for our work with STP. We believe that, during a LEGO® build, the hands provide a conduit through which the DMN and TPN can work their magic to build and create new stories of our world. The back-and-forth process, external-internal referencing, without our conscious internal dialogue or the use of verbal language, can reduce the interference of the DMN's current worldview required to see things afresh (see client quote earlier).

Chapter 1 discussed how developing our skills, thinking, and feeling are rooted in bodily experiences, particularly using hands. Chapter 2 introduced two important brain networks – the DMN and TPN – and how these networks underpin our understanding of how we take in and processes information – particularly via play. We presented a link between brain networks and how play can assist people to explore and develop new worldviews. Chapter 3 discusses the biology, evolution, and importance of play. We also introduce the notion of "serious play" and how social connection and play can build a deeper relationship with one's tribe.

References

Apter, M. (1997). Reversal theory: What is it? *Psychologist*, *10*, 217–220.

Atzil, S., Gao, W., Fradkin, I., & Barrett, L. F. (2018). Growing a social brain. *Nature Human Behaviour*, *2*(9), 624–636. https://doi.org/10.1038/s41562-018-0384-6

Barber, A. D., Caffo, B. S., Pekar, J. J., & Mostofsky, S. H. (2013). Developmental changes in within- and between-network connectivity between late childhood and adulthood. *Neuropsychologia, 51*(1), 156–167. https://doi.org/10.1016/j.neuropsychologia.2012.11.011

Baum, G. L., Cui, Z., Roalf, D. R., Ciric, R., Betzel, R. F., Larsen, B., Cieslak, M., Cook, P. A., Xia, C. H., Moore, T. M., Ruparel, K., Oathes, D. J., Alexander-Bloch, A. F., Shinohara, R. T., Raznahan, A., Gur, R. E., Gur, R. C., Bassett, D. S., & Satterthwaite, T. D. (2020). Development of structure-function coupling in human brain networks during youth. *Proceedings of the National Academy of Sciences, 117*(1), 771–778. https://doi.org/10.1073/pnas.1912034117

Beaty, R. E., Seli, P., & Schacter, D. L. (2019). Network neuroscience of creative cognition: Mapping cognitive mechanisms and individual differences in the creative brain. *Current Opinion in Behavioral Sciences, 27*, 22–30. https://doi.org/10.1016/j.cobeha.2018.08.013

Boyatzis, R. E., Rochford, K., & Jack, A. I. (2014). Antagonistic neural networks underlying differentiated leadership roles. *Frontiers in Human Neuroscience, 8*, 114. https://doi.org/10.3389/fnhum.2014.00114

Boyatzis, R. E., Rochford, K., & Taylor, S. N. (2015). The role of the positive emotional attractor in vision and shared vision: Toward effective leadership, relationships, and engagement. *Frontiers in Psychology, 6*. https://doi.org/10.3389/fpsyg.2015.00670

Camacho, M. C., Quiñones-Camacho, L. E., & Perlman, S. B. (2020). Does the child brain rest?: An examination and interpretation of resting cognition in developmental cognitive neuroscience. *NeuroImage, 212*, 116688. https://doi.org/10.1016/j.neuroimage.2020.116688

Chaddock-Heyman, L., Weng, T. B., Kienzler, C., Erickson, K. I., Voss, M. W., Drollette, E. S., Raine, L. B., Kao, S.-C., Hillman, C. H., & Kramer, A. F. (2018). Scholastic performance and functional connectivity of brain networks in children. *PLoS One, 13*(1). https://doi.org/10.1371/journal.pone.0190073

Cieri, F., & Esposito, R. (2019). Psychoanalysis and neuroscience: The bridge between mind and brain. *Frontiers in Psychology, 10*. www.frontiersin.org/article/10.3389/fpsyg.2019.01983

Csikszentmihalyi, M. (2008). *Flow: The psychology of optimal experience*. Harper Perennial.

Deming, P. (2021). *Large-scale brain networks in psychopathy* [PhD thesis, The University of Wisconsin]. www.proquest.com/docview/2544427437/abstract/821CEA60BA6249C1PQ/1

Dunbar, R. I. M., & Shultz, S. (2017). Why are there so many explanations for primate brain evolution? *Philosophical Transactions of the Royal Society B: Biological Sciences, 372*(1727), 20160244. https://doi.org/10.1098/rstb.2016.0244

Fuchs, E., & Flügge, G. (2014). Adult neuroplasticity: More than 40 years of research. *Neural Plasticity, 2014*, 1–10. https://doi.org/10.1155/2014/541870

Gopnik, A. (2011a). *The philosophical baby: What children's minds tell us about truth, love & the meaning of life*. Random House.

Gopnik, A. (Director). (2011b, July). *What do babies think?* www.ted.com/talks/alison_gopnik_what_do_babies_think

Gopnik, A. (2017, February 16). When children beat adults at seeing the world. *Wall Street Journal*. www.wsj.com/articles/when-children-beat-adults-at-seeing-the-world-1487266807

Gopnik, A. (2021, April 16). *Ezra Klein interviews Alison Gopnik* [Interview]. www.nytimes.com/2021/04/16/podcasts/ezra-klein-podcast-alison-gopnik-transcript.html

Hebb, D. O. (1949). *The organization of behavior; a neuropsychological theory* (pp. xix, 335). John Wiley & Sons.

Hughes, C., Cassidy, B. S., Faskowitz, J., Avena-Koenigsberger, A., Sporns, O., & Krendl, A. C. (2019). Age differences in specific neural connections within the default mode network underlie theory of mind. *NeuroImage, 191*, 269–277. https://doi.org/10.1016/j.neuroimage.2019.02.024

Krönke, K.-M., Wolff, M., Shi, Y., Kräplin, A., Smolka, M. N., Bühringer, G., & Goschke, T. (2020). Functional connectivity in a triple-network saliency model is associated with real-life self-control. *Neuropsychologia, 149*, 107667. https://doi.org/10.1016/j.neuropsychologia.2020.107667

Kucyi, A., Esterman, M., Riley, C. S., & Valera, E. M. (2016). Spontaneous default network activity reflects behavioral variability independent of mind-wandering. *Proceedings of the National Academy of Sciences, 113*(48), 13899–13904. https://doi.org/10.1073/pnas.1611743113

Li, W., Mai, X., & Liu, C. (2014). The default mode network and social understanding of others: What do brain connectivity studies tell us. *Frontiers in Human Neuroscience, 8*. https://doi.org/10.3389/fnhum.2014.00074

Liu, C., Solis, L., Jensen, H., Hopkins, E., Neale, D., Zosh, J., Hirsh-Pasek, K., & Whitebread, D. (2017). *Neuroscience and learning through play: A review of the evidence.* https://doi.org/10.13140/RG.2.2.11789.84963

Luu, P., Tucker, D. M., & Stripling, R. (2007). Neural mechanisms for learning actions in context. *Brain Research, 1179*, 89–105. https://doi.org/10.1016/j.brainres.2007.03.092

Maharjan, R., Diaz Bustamante, L., Ghattas, K. N., Ilyas, S., Al-Refai, R., & Khan, S. (2020). Role of lifestyle in neuroplasticity and neurogenesis in an aging brain. *Cureus, 12*(9), e10639. https://doi.org/10.7759/cureus.10639

Mars, R. B., Neubert, F.-X., Noonan, M. P., Sallet, J., Toni, I., & Rushworth, M. F. S. (2012). On the relationship between the "default mode network" and the "social brain". *Frontiers in Human Neuroscience, 6*. https://doi.org/10.3389/fnhum.2012.00189

Moran, J. M., Kelley, W. M., & Heatherton, T. F. (2013). What can the organization of the brain's default mode network tell us about self-knowledge? *Frontiers in Human Neuroscience, 7*. https://doi.org/10.3389/fnhum.2013.00391

Queensland Brain Institute. (2016, November 22). *Adult neurogenesis.* https://qbi.uq.edu.au/brain-basics/brain-physiology/adult-neurogenesis

Raichle, M. E. (2010). The brain's dark energy. *Scientific American, 302*(3), 44–49. https://doi.org/10.1038/scientificamerican0310-44

Raichle, M. E. (2015). The brain's default mode network. *Annual Review of Neuroscience, 38*(1), 433–447. https://doi.org/10.1146/annurev-neuro-071013-014030

Raichle, M. E., MacLeod, A. M., Snyder, A. Z., Powers, W. J., Gusnard, D. A., & Shulman, G. L. (2001). A default mode of brain function. *Proceedings of the National Academy of Sciences, 98*(2), 676–682. https://doi.org/10.1073/pnas.98.2.676

Rubinstein, D., & Lahad, M. (2022). Fantastic reality: The role of imagination, playfulness, and creativity in healing trauma. *Traumatology*. https://doi.org/10.1037/trm0000376

Ruckli, B. (2016). *The meaning of creative activities in the lives of people in remission of mental* [Doctoral thesis, University of Brighton]. https://research.brighton.ac.uk/files/4752116/Binder2.pdf

Sakai, J. (2020). Core concept: How synaptic pruning shapes neural wiring during development and, possibly, in disease. *Proceedings of the National Academy of Sciences, 117*(28), 16096–16099. https://doi.org/10.1073/pnas.2010281117

Smallwood, J., Bernhardt, B. C., Leech, R., Bzdok, D., Jefferies, E., & Margulies, D. S. (2021). The default mode network in cognition: A topographical perspective. *Nature Reviews Neuroscience, 22*(8), 503–513. https://doi.org/10.1038/s41583-021-00474-4

Smallwood, J., Gorgolewski, K. J., Golchert, J., Ruby, F. J. M., Engen, H., Baird, B., Vinski, M. T., Schooler, J. W., & Margulies, D. S. (2013). The default modes of reading: Modulation of posterior cingulate and medial prefrontal cortex connectivity associated with comprehension and task focus while reading. *Frontiers in Human Neuroscience, 7*, 734. https://doi.org/10.3389/fnhum.2013.00734

Smallwood, J., Turnbull, A., Wang, H., Ho, N. S. P., Poerio, G. L., Karapanagiotidis, T., Konu, D., Mckeown, B., Zhang, M., Murphy, C., Vatansever, D., Bzdok, D., Konishi, M., Leech, R., Seli, P., Schooler, J. W., Bernhardt, B., Margulies, D. S., & Jefferies, E. (2021). The neural correlates of ongoing conscious thought. *IScience, 24*(3), 102132. https://doi.org/10.1016/j.isci.2021.102132

Spreng, R. N. (2012). The fallacy of a "task-negative" network. *Frontiers in Psychology, 3*. https://doi.org/10.3389/fpsyg.2012.00145

Sun, J., Liu, Z., Rolls, E. T., Chen, Q., Yao, Y., Yang, W., Wei, D., Zhang, Q., Zhang, J., Feng, J., & Qiu, J. (2019). Verbal creativity correlates with the temporal variability of brain networks during the resting state. *Cerebral Cortex, 29*(3), 1047–1058. https://doi.org/10.1093/cercor/bhy010

Takeuchi, H., Taki, Y., Nouchi, R., Sekiguchi, A., Hashizume, H., Sassa, Y., Kotozaki, Y., Miyauchi, C. M., Yokoyama, R., Iizuka, K., Nakagawa, S., Nagase, T., Kunitoki, K., & Kawashima, R. (2013). Resting state functional connectivity associated with trait emotional intelligence. *NeuroImage, 83*, 318–328. https://doi.org/10.1016/j.neuroimage.2013.06.044

Tylén, K., Christensen, P., Roepstorff, A., Lund, T., Østergaard, S., & Donald, M. (2015). Brains striving for coherence: Long-term cumulative plot formation in the default mode network. *NeuroImage*, *121*, 106–114. https://doi.org/10.1016/j.neuroimage.2015.07.047

van Elk, M., Arciniegas Gomez, M. A., van der Zwaag, W., van Schie, H. T., & Sauter, D. (2019). The neural correlates of the awe experience: Reduced default mode network activity during feelings of awe. *Human Brain Mapping*, *40*(12), 3561–3574. https://doi.org/10.1002/hbm.24616

Witt, S. T., van Ettinger-Veenstra, H., Salo, T., Riedel, M. C., & Laird, A. R. (2021). *What executive function network is that? An image-based meta-analysis of network labels*. https://doi.org/10.1101/2020.07.14.201202

Wright, J. J., Wright, S., Sadlo, G., & Stew, G. (2014). A reversal theory exploration of flow process and the flow channel. *Journal of Occupational Science*, *21*(2), 188–201. https://doi.org/10.1080/14427591.2012.713313

Zosh, J. M., Hirsh-Pasek, K., Hopkins, E. J., Jensen, H., Liu, C., Neale, D., Solis, S. L., & Whitebread, D. (2018). Accessing the inaccessible: Redefining play as a spectrum. *Frontiers in Psychology*, *9*, 1124. https://doi.org/10.3389/fpsyg.2018.01124

CHAPTER 3
THE BIOLOGY AND EVOLUTION OF PLAY

Alec Hamilton

Chapter 3 centres on understanding human play's biological and evolutionary purpose. While play is ubiquitous, its definition is often viewed as "ambiguous, variable, and elusive" (Demanchick & Peabody, 2015, p. 407). Despite the challenges faced in defining play, it is well captured by the following description:

> a phenomenon of life that everyone is acquainted with firsthand. . . . Familiarity with play is more than merely individual; it is a collective, public familiarity. Play is a well-known and common fact of the social world . . . it is always an occurrence that is luminously *suffused with sense* [sinnhaft], an enactment that is experienced. We live in the enjoyment of the act of play (which, mind you, pre-supposes no reflexive self-consciousness). . . . For the adult, . . . play is a strange oasis, a dreamy resting point. . . . Play gives us the present.
>
> (Fink, 1957/2016, pp. 15, 21)

The chapter focuses primarily on human play and blurs the line between "pure-play" and the use of play within the context of its therapeutic application. The line between play and its therapeutic application is blurred because many definitions require play to be the goal "in of itself." "Play

DOI: 10.4324/9781003260424-4

is the antithesis of work or serious behaviour" (Bateson & Martin, 2013, p. 12). The challenge here is that therapeutic play can be fun but has a purpose, is often serious, and can involve negative emotions. Therefore, we will describe what we mean by "Serious Play" within the context of Seriously Therapeutic Play with LEGO® (STP) and how this blurring of the definition of play stays within the broader context of play; namely, playfulness.

Play and playfulness

Play is viewed as a physical or mental act or experience that many agree needs to be voluntary and intrinsically rewarding, while playfulness is seen as a cognitive behavioural attribute – a "state of mind in which an individual can think flexibly, take risks with ideas (or interactions), and allow creative thoughts to emerge" (Youell, 2008, p. 122).

Youell argues that playfulness

- Happens in a relationship.
- Is an essential aspect of play.
- Is an important factor in teaching and learning.
- Play and work are not opposites or mutually exclusive; for example, play is work for babies and young children.

Playfulness has been further defined as a positive mood state "and allows people to frame or reframe everyday situations in a way such that they experience them as entertaining, and/or intellectually stimulating, and/or personally interesting" (Proyer et al., 2019, p. 46). Being playful at work is reported to have many benefits, reducing stress and increasing creativity and innovation (Proyer et al., 2019). Our premise is that playfulness is the bridge between play and our notion of serious play. Demanchick and Peabody (2015) point out that "play therapy" or "play as therapy" requires a purposeful or serious approach within a therapeutic relationship; this is "serious play" – play as a state of mind and disposition – i.e., playfulness. In serious play, one can be purposefully playful, take risks, develop ideas, interact constructively, experience negative and positive emotions, build relationships, and work towards change.

Does play have a biological and evolutionary purpose?

In 1901, Karl Groos (1901/2018, pp. 2, 3) wrote that higher animals are born with "natural or hereditary impulse" that produce "activity without serious intent . . . 'play'." These biological impulses drive a child to explore their environment, imitate the behaviours of others, build their understanding of the world, and develop the mental, emotional, and musculoskeletal capacities necessary for survival. Gray (2019) builds a modern-day picture of Groos' theory of play and its evolutionary importance through a modern research lens. They highlight a range of studies examining the behaviours observed in juvenile animal play and how they reflected adult behaviour. Gray proposes that play is a crucial aspect of learning:

> Humans are the cultural animal and, as such, are, by nature, the educative animal. Beginning at least 2 million years ago, early humans began moving along an evolutionary track that made them ever more dependent on education. . . . Children who failed to acquire crucial aspects of their culture would be at a serious survival and reproductive disadvantage, so natural selection would strongly favour characteristics that promoted children's desires and abilities to acquire the culture.
>
> (Gray, pp. 90–91)

More specifically, curiosity drives children to acquire knowledge, and play is how they acquire skills to gain that knowledge (interview with Peter Gray, Mehta et al., 2020).

In our everyday lives, we can observe many playful interactions between a parent and child, and if we scratch the surface, we can see how play is a mechanism by which the child can take in the world, explore, discover, and learn. We can observe young children playfully exploring the boundaries of their world and the boundaries their parents have drawn. This playful behaviour is a "mediator of change" (Demanchick & Peabody, 2015, p. 410), assisting in the development of culturally valued motor coordination, survival strategies and language (fighting, cooking, hunting, building, creating fire, etc.). Play also provides the opportunity for children to explore emotional experiences. Children play with their emotions; they "play" at being scared, take risks, fail, and try again. They learn resilience and how to manage their anxieties. Play is a child's work; their "serious play" ensures their survival by learning the social norms and what is culturally significant. Gray (2019) comments that, in the past few decades, there has been a noticeable reduction in children's risky play and, interestingly, a "well-documented increase in anxiety and decline in emotional resilience" (p. 93). This is certainly something I have observed in my psychological practice.

The notion that, for babies and children, play is work resonates with Gopnik's (2017) description of Spotlight and Lantern attention (discussed in Chapter 2). Gopnik suggests that a critical difference between children and adults is the focus of their attention. It is a biological imperative for children to take in an explorative view of the world, a lantern view, which is wide open and diverse; they "playfully explore" to make sense, and ultimately, learn about the world. On the other hand, adults focus their attention like a spotlight; it is goal-directed; they take what they know, building on this knowledge to help them exploit their environment to survive. While adults play and are playful, their attention is focussed. When adults play and are playful, they tend to aim for fun, and interestingly, this playfulness is often a time of creativity and innovation – as it is for children. Gray (2019) also suggests that adult play is often associated with the concept of "flow" (Csikszentmihalyi, 2008), which Gray describes as a "state of mind" consistent with a playful disposition.

Babies in play

I recently became a grandparent of twin girls. It has been fascinating to watch them "work at playing" with their environment. I watched how they initially took in their environment with their eyes, then through their mouths, and now they explore with their bodies. They are naturally playful, and it seems, from the outside, that they are, in fact, extremely goal focussed. Their "work" is seriously playful. Through their playful behaviour and interactions, they have gained connections with themselves, each other, their parents, and their wider world. Child development explains the biological basis of my grandchildren's playful introduction to their world. Being a grandparent and watching twins is fascinating, as their development occurs more overtly in front of your eyes: one child starts a new skill, and the other soon follows. While my training in child development makes me acutely aware that they are learning through play, their development seems so miraculous – it's just so amazing to watch it in stereo. I keep falling into wonder – why did one behaviour develop now, and why not a day or an hour ago? Why can't they do something a day later but can then do it the next day?

We know the answer to why their playful work lies in our evolutionary past. Developmentally, it makes perfect sense that a baby's initial eye focus should be about 20–25 cm from their face, roughly the distance between the baby and their mother's face while breastfeeding. I have been able to observe two young beings respond to their mother by turning their heads when she touches their cheek. Their sucking and rooting reflex facilitated their attachment and feeding. It seems fascinating that, as their gaze expands, they learn to interact with their hands and use them as toys and pacifiers. The twins experience joy at discovering their hands time and time again. I've observed how the grasping reflex has helped the girls grasp for safety and play. It is exciting to hear a cousin exclaim, "She held my hand!" after placing their finger in the girl's palm.

Now we see the girls starting to play with their "voice," gurgling and cooing. Their personalities are emerging, and they are each developing in their own way; one blew "raspberries" while the other giggled. The girls are now skilled at interacting with one initiating and the other responding; they have started playing peek-a-boo by themselves; and they have definitely moved to dropping food from their highchairs, laughing at each other, and engaging with their parent's reactions.

The biology behind social interaction

Writing in COVID-19 times has been interesting from a biological and evolutionary perspective. Many years have passed since our societies have come under pressure from global pandemics, wars, or disasters. We have experienced unprecedented levels of isolation resulting from lockdowns and quarantine. This has resulted in a broader interest in the influencing factors behind mental health issues like depression and anxiety due to our societal responses to the COVID-19 pandemic. Why has this level of isolation – this loss of *connection* – significantly affected our mental health?

It has become evident during the COVID-19 pandemic quarantining, lockdowns, and isolations that humans have an instinctual and significant need to be connected socially. Human beings are biologically driven to be social animals. It became clear that online connections, the only method available during lockdowns, could not mediate the loss of physical human-to-human contact. In a review of the literature on the psychological impact of quarantine undertaken by Brooks et al. (2020), the authors indicated that those who had been quarantined reported high levels of psychological distress: "emotional disturbance, depression, stress, low mood, irritability, insomnia, posttraumatic stress symptoms anger, and emotional exhaustion, low mood and irritability . . . avoidance behaviours and consideration of resignation" (p. 913).

Negative responses were also reported from those close contacts who were also required to quarantine. The studies that reported comparison data between those quarantined and the general population all reported an increase in psychological distress in those quarantined, compared to those who have not been. One study said that "post-traumatic stress scores were four times higher in children who had been quarantined" (p. 913). Ganesan et al. (2021), in their summary of the impact of COVID-19 on mental health and suicide, indicate that "with social distancing, isolation, and lockdown, people may suffer from very serious psychological issues, such as anxiety, stress, fear, fear-induced overreactive behaviour, frustration, guilt, anger, boredom, sadness, worry, nervousness, helplessness, loneliness, insomnia, and depression" (p. 3).

In a systematic review focusing on the impact of quarantine on children and adolescents, Imran et al. (2020) reported that, while there is a "lack of conclusive evidence of the impact of quarantine and isolation on children and adolescents," isolation, social exclusion stigma, and fear appear to be common outcomes (p. 1106). "Children and adolescents need to stay connected with family and friends, which gets difficult with school closures, limited visits with friends and families etc. Inability to activate your social network is noted to be associated with anxiety and distress" (p. 1112). Lee (2020) indicates that 1.5 billion children were out of school at one point in the pandemic. The routines and social interaction within the school environment provide an anchor for many students, and this anchor is often the cornerstone in supporting mental health. The effect on younger students is also of great concern as the evidence suggests they may be particularly impacted by school closures and lockdowns, with 4–10-year-olds, reported to have "pronounced changes in their pro-social functioning" (McNeill & Gillon, 2021, p. 3) and missing the crucial social experiences we would typically see. Pre-adolescents, in particular, are "suffering more" than older students (Almeida et al., 2021, p. 3). COVID-19 isolation limited physical and social interaction; students could not spend time with friends, playgrounds were closed, and people feared spending time outside their homes. Gray (cited in Mehta et al., 2020) connects the rise in mental health issues with the decrease in young people's opportunity to play, commenting that "a third of school-aged children are suffering from a clinically significant anxiety disorder and at least 20% are suffering from depression . . . [and] the rate of mental health admissions for school children is double during the school year, than when it is off" (p. 687) when children are not in the structured environment of school and able to play.

Social communication and brain development

Robin Dunbar (1993), in their seminal work on the evolution of language and social groups, commented that "primates are, above all, social animals . . . [however] animals cannot maintain the cohesion and integrity of groups larger than a size fixed by the information-processing capacity of their neocortex" (p. 681). The connections maintained in primate groups are influenced by the time involved in grooming behaviour. Social grooming behaviour builds and reinforces the group's social connections – "friendships." The amount of time spent in social grooming correlates with the group's size; "more grooming = larger group size." However, the group size relates more to the strength of connection within the friendship groups. Connected individuals are shielded from harassment and stress, and the number of smaller, connected groups influences the total group size. How does this relate to *homo sapiens* – to us today? To answer this, Dunbar investigated the link between group and neocortical size. They propose that, while grooming and the associated motor-neural development build the depth of social connection, there is also an association between language development and successful group coherence strategy for maintaining connection within larger modern human groups.

Social grooming requires time. Larger groups required more grooming to maintain group connections. At a specific size, the group's members would simply run out of enough time to groom the individuals within a larger social group. If group size is to grow, other mechanisms must be developed to maintain and develop the more complex connections within the group. Through the analysis of a range of anthropological studies, Dunbar reported that modern human group size sat within three distinct sizes:

- Small, living groups (30–50 individuals).
- Large population unit, tribe (200–2500 individuals).
- The culturally connected clan (100–200 people) with a group size of around 150, the functional limit of a connected group of individuals.

To maintain the connections required in a group of 150 individuals, Dunbar calculated that they would need to spend about 40% of their time grooming – more than double that seen in any nonhuman primate group. There is simply not enough time in the day to groom at this level, find food, sleep, and maintain the connections vital to group cohesion.

The social brain hypothesis (Dunbar & Shultz, 2017) emphasises that a group of animals' ability to build strong social-relational connections is crucial to developing and maintaining increasingly larger coherent and connected groups. Dunbar hypothesised that brain growth and language development formed the mechanism by which group size could be increased without reliance on grooming behaviour. "Language evolved as a 'cheap' form of social grooming, thereby enabling the ancestral humans to maintain the cohesion of the unusually large groups" (1993, p. 689). "There is now extensive evidence that social network size and quality are among the most important factors influencing health, well being and even longevity in humans" (2017, p. 6). Living in groups creates stress, and, as we have seen recently, being removed physically from our clan also increases stress. The ability to manage social connections, both those direct and those indirect or absent relationships (Zoom friendships), is cognitively demanding and forms the basis for our ability (or inability) to keep others in mind and infer their thinking (Theory of Mind). "Not only do individuals' mentalising abilities correlate with the size of their social networks in humans, but they also correlate with the volume of core regions in the brain, especially in the prefrontal cortex and the temporal lobes" (p. 9).

Play that builds connection: the clan in action

As a school psychologist, I watch year after year students of all ages (and teachers) trying to find their clan. Belonging to the clan has tremendous attraction and power over the individual – highly evident in high school social groups. We see and hear about the negative side of school clans; however, there are many examples of the positive influences of school sport, drama, and music clans.

Music camp: music is play

One of the most enlightening school trips I have been on in my nearly 40-year professional career was a week-long, year-9 music camp. I was lucky to be "roped in" as the bus driver. It was a simple role: drive them from place to place, then get out of the way as the group organised themselves and their equipment.

I was an observer of a world I had never participated in before. I have taken many students on camp but never in this essential, perfunctory role. For the first time, I had the privilege of observing the joy of a middle school clan without any of the "normal" drama and angst. A clan that came together just for this adventure, a group that seriously played together; they played at making music, played via impromptu signing, and played physical and language-based games. The group were clearly aware of the times they needed to be serious and perform. These serious play times were times for creativity, joy, and playing together. They came together as an orchestra, a band, a duo, and as teachers of younger students. They were contextually playful with each other, the students they met, and the adults they performed for in the aged care facilities. They were also very playful with each other outside these more serious times.

I witnessed their absolute joy at being together for no other purpose than to bring their music and joy to semi-remote communities. The connections this quite disparate group of students and their teachers made with each other and their audience through making music was phenomenal. The spontaneous signing on the bus and the vibrancy and positivity in their formal and informal conversation seem consistent with a clan building itself through their shared language and play. The group "maintained its cohesion" through song, serious play, and the social structures they collectively created. It was the first camp I have ever been on that didn't have to assign a naughty student to clean the bus. Firstly, there wasn't any rubbish, and secondly, no student misbehaved. I never heard a cross word or a teacher's lecture during our time together. I had experienced how "music is play for everyone" (Brown, 2020).

Handball: building social skills

One of the great joys of playground duty is watching the social development of Grade 2 and 3 students through the game of handball (also called down-ball or four square [n square]; see https://en.wikipedia. org/wiki/Handball_(schoolyard_game)). Every year, I spend a fair amount of time supporting children in successfully managing conflict with their peers as they start to build their clan, particularly via handball. In my school, handball has high social status; therefore, some students need to be successful, as a tremendous amount of social power comes from that success. Handball involves a group of students hitting a ball at each other. Each student stands on the court in a square and tries to get another student out of their square. The squares are numbered from king downwards, depending on the number of squares or players. The aim is to be king and protect yourself. If you are not the king, you aim to maintain your status and get the king out. There are a set of defined rules generally based around the king serving the ball by bouncing it in their square first and hitting it with their hand, so it bounces in their opponent's square. The opponents must return the serve or direct the ball to another opponent.

From this basic starting point, things become complex because, as each group develops, they build their own unique set of rules. We find that the clan has emerged about halfway through the year, and membership has been established through play. About this time, the Grade 2 and 3 (about 7 years of age) students start to develop their own rules, and things become interesting. This occurs in a few different ways, with clan members declaring "ball owner's rules," "collective rules," or the "loudest, strongest, most volatile student's rules." At the same time, we also see the emergence of the students "theory of mind" with the students starting to understand nuance, lies, and white lies and social faux pas (Osterhaus & Koerber, 2021). We begin to see stronger peer relationships and peer group power. The importance of social dynamics becomes prominent, and we see conflict increase. The students build their own clan rules, and those with social handball status and the ability to adapt and change with the changing rules exercise their authority over the game and each other.

The confluence of brain and social development, social power, flexibility/rigidity of thinking, and social influence combine to create a rich social dynamic. As a psychologist, handball provides a rich social development experience and an opportunity for conflict resolution. As an administrator, handball becomes a game of continued peer conflict, with day-after-day emotional outbursts, arguments, and altercations. Inevitably, late in the term, a member of the administration has had enough, and they step in, posting *the rules* and providing more supervision. At this point, many students shift away from the game to other social play, which is consistent with Gray's comments on the negative influence adults have when they over structure children's play and how these actions curb the children's "natural drive to play" (as cited in Mehta et al., 2020, p. 687).

In the last 2 or so years, during and after the COVID-19 school closure and lockdowns, I have noticed a significant change in the development of social groups in Grade 2 and Grade 3 students. My interest was initially captured by the apparent quietness of the playground and fewer children asking for my help managing conflict. I was simply not as busy with handball conflict. Term 3 came and went without the administration having to post the rules, and the handball courts had other games being played, and there was a reduction in those sitting and waiting to join. I followed up with some students and asked what they were playing. Most played "chasey" (tag, https://en.wikipedia.org/wiki/Tag_ (game)). Chasey has few rules; one person is "it," and the "it" person runs around catching others, so they become "it" or join the "it group."

The game changes its name depending on the current social theme, but the rules remain the same. Chasey has little conflict, and when it arises, it generally occurs when someone feels targeted, is not "going out" when caught, or always playing "their" game. The conflict seems to be individual 1:1 and personal. Chasey has less social structure than handball, is perhaps more equal, and therefore doesn't specifically help the children develop conflict resolution skills. The playground has more movement and sweaty children but less conflict. I'm not seeing the establishment of a strong peer group. I'm seeing a more collective sense of group but perhaps fewer close connections between the players. Children seem to be running around without connecting to the game or each other. I'm also not seeing the depth of relationships or the same level of social connection. There is less of a sense of clan. When I mentioned this to the teachers, they commented that, while there is less peer conflict, they have also noticed a lack of cohesion in their classes.

Conclusion

The music camp, Chasey, and handball are examples of activities that provided an opportunity for play which can "significantly predict both social success and individual adaptability" (Greve & Thomsen, 2016). These observations are also consistent with evolutionary biologists' belief about the importance of play (see LaFreniere, 2011). Chasey and handball have elements of play that help children build physical skills – running, hand-eye coordination, balance, and sense of body in space. These forms of play allowed the students to acquire a range of cultural skills and values and assisted them in learning how to build friendships, connect with peers, control their emotions, and refine their problem-solving skills. The language used in negotiating handball rules is consistent with a group "grooming" itself, developing its social norms and establishing the social conventions of the clan. The students' success at managing handball conflict was consistent with Greve and Thomsen's findings of a positive relationship between adaptability, play and social success. Chasey's lack of language and interaction seems consistent with my observation of less cohesion and sense of clan. Chasey's lack of apparent social connection would suggest this is less valuable for social cohesion and adaptability than handball.

The formal nature of the music camp, whilst more structured, provided an opportunity for skill development that was more age and context-appropriate. The camp had a great sense of playfulness with the students' spontaneous signing and being playful with each other and their audiences. The more adaptable the student to the rules, the more success in managing conflict and, it would seem from my observations, greater social status. The greater the opportunity for play that utilises language to build and groom the clan, the greater social cohesion.

The COVID pandemic took away or, at the very least, limited students' social interaction. The venues for building social skills and group cohesion were simply removed. In Melbourne, Australia, for example, 5 million people were locked down for 262 days, the longest in the world (Al Jazeera, 2021). At the time of writing this chapter, it was early in the post-pandemic period. While the research points at some difficult days ahead for students and adults alike, it also appears younger children may be more affected by the lockdowns, separation anxiety has increased, and their social skills are lagging (Adams, 2022; Hall, 2022). The three school activities reported earlier show how group cohesion and the human need for connection are mediated through play. The music clan seemed to build itself spontaneously, vibrantly, and dynamically through playing music and their playfulness. While just as spontaneous, handball was often vibrant in a different, perhaps slightly negative, way. Yet, it still created opportunities for positive conflict and the development of the clan's norms and social structure. Chasey also provides the opportunity for connection, but it appears less attuned to developing broader or generalised group cohesion. Without too much adult involvement, the music camp, handball, and Chasey are all involved in building a social structure with cultural and social advantages. Those activities that create stronger connections provide more significant social advantage.

References

Adams, R. (2022, May 17). Younger children most affected by COVID lockdowns, new research finds. *The Guardian*. www.theguardian.com/education/2022/may/18/younger-children-most-affected-by-covid-lockdowns-new-research-finds

Al Jazeera. (2021, October 17). Melbourne set to bring an end to world's longest lockdowns. *Al Jazeera*. www.aljazeera.com/news/2021/10/17/australias-melbourne-set-to-end-worlds-longest-lockdowns

Almeida, M., Challa, M., Ribeiro, M., Harrison, A. M., & Castro, M. C. (2021). Editorial perspective: The mental health impact of school closures during the COVID-19 pandemic. *Journal of Child Psychology and Psychiatry, and Allied Disciplines*. https://doi.org/10.1111/jcpp.13535

Bateson, P. P. G., & Martin, P. (2013). The biology of play. In *Play, playfulness, creativity and innovation* (pp. 10–27). Cambridge University Press. eBook Collection (EBSCOhost). https://search.ebscohost.com/login.aspx?direct=true&db=nlebk&AN=592754&site=ehost-live&authtype=ip,sso&custid=s9679029

Brooks, S. K., Webster, R. K., Smith, L. E., Woodland, L., Wessely, S., Greenberg, N., & Rubin, G. J. (2020). The psychological impact of quarantine and how to reduce it: Rapid review of the evidence. *The Lancet*, *395*(10227), 912–920. https://doi.org/10.1016/S0140-6736(20)30460-8

Brown, S. (2020). Music is play for everyone. *PlayCore*. www.playcore.com/news/music-is-play-for-everyone

Csikszentmihalyi, M. (2008). *Flow: The psychology of optimal experience*. Harper Perennial.

Demanchick, S. P., & Peabody, M. A. (2015). Play therapy on the edge: Understanding definitions and change mechanisms. In J. E. Johnson, S. G. Eberle, T. S. Henricks, & D. Kuschner (Eds.), *The handbook of the study of play*. Rowman & Littlefield.

Dunbar, R. I. M. (1993). Coevolution of neocortical size, group size and language in humans. *Behavioral and Brain Sciences*, *16*(4), 681–694. https://doi.org/10.1017/S0140525X00032325

Dunbar, R. I. M., & Shultz, S. (2017). Why are there so many explanations for primate brain evolution? *Philosophical Transactions of the Royal Society B: Biological Sciences*, *372*(1727), 20160244. https://doi.org/10.1098/rstb.2016.0244

Fink, E. (2016). Oasis of happiness: Thoughts toward an ontology of play. In *Play as symbol of the world: And other writings*. Indiana University Press. eBook Collection (EBSCOhost). https://search.ebscohost.com/login.aspx?direct=true&db=nlebk&AN=1252180&site=ehost-live&authtype=ip,sso&custid=s9679029 (Original work published 1957)

Ganesan, B., Al-Jumaily, A., Fong, K. N. K., Prasad, P., Meena, S. K., & Tong, R. K.-Y. (2021). Impact of coronavirus disease 2019 (Covid-19) outbreak quarantine, isolation, and lockdown policies on mental health and suicide. *Frontiers in Psychiatry*, *12*, 565190. https://doi.org/10.3389/fpsyt.2021.565190

Gopnik, A. (2017, February 16). When children beat adults at seeing the world. *Wall Street Journal*. www.wsj.com/articles/when-children-beat-adults-at-seeing-the-world-1487266807

Gray, P. (2019). Evolutionary functions of play: Practice, resilience, innovation, and cooperation. In P. K. Smith & J. Roopnarine (Eds.), *The Cambridge handbook of play: Developmental and disciplinary perspectives* (pp. 84–102). Cambridge University Press. https://cdn2.psychologytoday.com/assets/evol.functs.play_published.pdf

Greve, W., & Thomsen, T. (2016). Evolutionary advantages of free play during childhood. *Evolutionary Psychology, 14*(4), 1474704916675349. https://doi.org/10.1177/1474704916675349

Groos, K. (2018). *The play of man* (E. Baldwin, Trans.; The Project Gutenberg). www.gutenberg.org/files/58411/58411-h/58411-h.htm#Page_1 (Original work published 1901)

Hall, R. (2022, April 4). "Empathy isn't there": The pandemic effects on children's social skills. *The Guardian*. www.theguardian.com/uk-news/2022/apr/04/empathy-isnt-there-the-pandemic-effects-on-childrens-social-skills

Imran, N., Aamer, I., Sharif, M. I., Bodla, Z. H., & Naveed, S. (2020). Psychological burden of quarantine in children and adolescents: A rapid systematic review and proposed solutions. *Pakistan Journal of Medical Sciences, 36*(5), 1106–1116. https://doi.org/10.12669/pjms.36.5.3088

LaFreniere, P. (2011). Evolutionary functions of social play. *American Journal of Play, 3*(4), 25.

Lee, J. (2020). Mental health effects of school closures during COVID-19. *The Lancet: Child & Adolescent Health, 4*(6), 421. https://doi.org/10.1016/S2352-4642(20)30109-7

McNeill, B., & Gillon, G. T. (2021). Lockdown experiences of 10–13 year olds in New Zealand. *New Zealand Journal of Educational Studies*, 1–17. https://doi.org/10.1007/s40841-021-00237-w

Mehta, R., Henriksen, D., Mishra, P., & Deep-Play Research Group. (2020). "Let children play!": Connecting evolutionary psychology and creativity with Peter Gray. *TechTrends, 64*(5), 684–689. https://doi.org/10.1007/s11528-020-00535-y

Osterhaus, C., & Koerber, S. (2021). The development of advanced theory of mind in middle childhood: A longitudinal study from age 5 to 10 years. *Child Development, 92*(5), 1872–1888. https://doi.org/10.1111/cdev.13627

Proyer, R. T., Tandler, N., & Brauer, K. (2019). Playfulness and creativity: A selective review. In S. R. Luria, J. Baer, & J. C. Kaufman (Eds.), *Creativity and humor* (pp. 43–60). Academic Press. https://doi.org/10.1016/B978-0-12-813802-1.00002-8

Youell, B. (2008). The importance of play and playfulness. *European Journal of Psychotherapy & Counselling, 10*(2), 121–129. https://doi.org/10.1080/13642530802076193

Chapter 4
Psychology at play

Kristen Klassen

When using Seriously Therapeutic Play and playing with LEGO®, we ask participants not to think and to simply allow their hands to choose the bricks they need (if you have ever done a LEGO® SERIOUS PLAY® workshop, you might have heard the phrase "don't have a meeting with yourself!"). Participants and clients are almost always successful with this instruction; yet how do your hands *know* you need *that* transparent, blue 2x2 brick to effectively express your metaphor? (Of course, we are not so naive as to believe that it is indeed your hands that are thinking!) This chapter explores the psychological factors at play in STP that allow individuals to invest fully in the method as well as to benefit therapeutically. We begin with a broad understanding of play, move to a narrower definition of play therapy, then discuss the relevant psychological factors in STP, such as the development of psychological safety through experiential methods, the experience of flow, the advantage of the common third, and therapeutic presence.

What is play? (And what is not?)

Play is so fundamental to human development that the United Nations has enshrined it as a human right. Article 31 of the United Nations Convention on the Rights of the Child (1989) states that "every child has the right to rest and leisure, to engage in play and recreational activities appropriate to the age of the child and to participate freely in cultural life and the arts." Furthermore, many organisations have emerged to support and promote this fundamental human right, such as the International Play Association and the Right to Play. Although play is typically discussed and applied in the context of children, research continues to expound on the benefits of play and play-based therapies for all ages (Frey, 2015; Schaefer, 2003). Brown (2009) states that, as humans, we are meant to play throughout life, whether it is through art, music, physical activity, or social interaction. Research continually supports the position that play is the most advanced process for promoting individual development and social integration throughout the species. The role of play in individual development is detailed in Chapter 2, whereas the social component of play is discussed in Chapter 10.

While there is a clear understanding of the value of play, with respect to what activities or behaviours are actually encompassed by the word "play," there is less clarity. Schaefer and Drewes (2014) argue that play is defined by the presence of eight distinctive characteristics. The authors contend that any activity can be defined as play provided it is (1) freely chosen, (2) intrinsically motivated, and (3) personally directed by the player(s). To fall into the category of play, there must be (4) active involvement, with (5) pretence or non-literality, and (6) flexibility. Additionally, the activity or activities must (7) value means over ends and (8) involve multiple positive affects. However, this approach to defining play encompasses so many activities, many authors argue it is easier to discuss what is *not* play. Nachmanovitch (2009) argues that the opposite of play is not work, but instead, an approach of one-dimensionality or literal-mindedness, whereas Brown (2009) contends that the opposite of play is depression. What is or is not play, or on the opposite end of the play spectrum, is of less importance than what these analogies and explanations are alluding to: that play is more about a frame of mind or *psychological state*.

Defining play therapy

In alignment with our challenges to defining play itself, play therapy is similarly difficult to delineate. Virginia Axline, one of the pioneers of non-directive play therapy, defines the process simply as "an opportunity that is offered to the child to experience growth under the most favourable conditions" (1947, p. 12). Garry Landreth, a leader in Child-Centered Play Therapy (CCPT), adds that play is

> a dynamic interpersonal relationship between a child (or person of any age) and an individual trained in play therapy procedures who provides selected play materials and facilitates the development of a safe relationship for the [person] to fully express and explore self (feelings, thoughts, experiences, and behaviours) through play.
>
> (2012, p. 11)

The Association for Play Therapy definition extends the explanation to address approaches to play therapy and therapeutic outcomes; "the systematic use of a theoretical model to establish an interpersonal process wherein trained play therapists use the therapeutic powers of play to help clients prevent or resolve psychosocial difficulties and achieve optimal growth and development" (www.a4pt.org). The therapeutic powers of play referred to in this definition are numerous but are broadly categorised into four key domains: facilitating communication, fostering emotional wellness, increasing personal strengths, and enhancing social relationships (Schaefer & Drewes, 2014) (these concepts are also further developed in Chapter 9 in the context of the therapeutic factors necessary for change). What all of these definitions of play therapy hold in congruence is the use of relationship to facilitate the development of the individual through a fun and actively involving process.

Defining serious play

Serious Play as a concept came to awareness in the late 1990s and early 2000s and is an approach to learning, problem-solving, and innovation that involves the use of game-like processes, simulations, or other forms of play to engage people in creative and collaborative activities with a serious purpose (Schrage, 2000). Serious play can take many forms, including role-playing exercises, board games, video games, or other immersive simulations that require participants to use their imagination, creativity, and problem-solving skills to achieve specific objectives. The purpose or primary goal of serious play is to make learning and problem-solving in industry-specific contexts more engaging, enjoyable, and effective by tapping into people's natural tendencies to learn through play; through exploration, experimentation, and social interaction. However, serious play differs from play and play therapy in terms of its primary purpose and goals. Play may not or may not have any purpose beyond engagement and enjoyment, whereas play therapy focuses on emotional wellness and development. By contrast, serious play is intentionally designed to achieve specific learning or problem-solving objectives, and therefore, inherently violates one of the eight characteristics of play highlighted by Schaefer and Drewes (2014). Serious play has an objective or intention and values ends over means (Statler et al., 2011). Another key difference is that serious play is typically facilitated by trained professionals who guide the participants through the play activity, monitor their progress, and provide feedback and support as needed. By comparison, play activities may be unsupervised, and in play therapy, the therapist takes a more active role in helping the child process their emotions and work through their challenges (Kottman, 2011). While play and play therapy focus on emotional and social development, serious play focuses on achieving specific objectives through collaborative problem-solving and learning.

Drawing from these three definitions, play, play therapy, and serious play, we highlight the components pulled from each that are necessary for the effective implementation of Seriously Therapeutic Play: psychological state, relationship, and intention and, of course, all while maintaining the element of fun.

Psychological state

Safety

Despite the integral nature of psychological safety in therapeutic settings, the concept is usually discussed in the context of industry and work performance. As early as 1990, Kahn defined psychological safety as an individual's "sense of being able to show and employ oneself without fear of negative consequences to self-image, status or career" (p. 705). Kahn (1990) argued that people need to feel that the context or situation is trustworthy and secure and that there are clear expectations surrounding behaviour and consequences; in the absence of psychological safety, workers will disengage.

More recently, Google examined the role of psychological safety within the context of what makes teams operate most effectively. The researchers involved in the project initially hypothesised that factors such as group dynamics, individual skill sets, personality traits, and emotional intelligence would be most predictive of team efficacy. What they found was that, within these domains, psychological safety was consistently the most predictive. Additional researchers (Kim et al., 2020) have furthered this finding, suggesting that, in industry, high levels of psychological safety are associated with more satisfied and engaged employees who are encouraged to take more risks and benefit from more creative breakthroughs.

In the context of "knowing what we don't know," Adam Grant (2021) argues that, when psychological safety is present, employees perceive mistakes as opportunities to learn rather than threats to their career progression. Furthermore, not only are employees willing to take risks and fail, but they are also willing to openly share their struggles, as opposed to only stressing their strengths and successes. Dr Sue Johnson (2008) furthers this position, arguing that curiosity, openness to new experiences, and flexibility in beliefs emerge from feeling psychologically safe, whereas rigidity and vigilance to threats materialise when safety is absent.

In the therapeutic context, psychological safety is essential for clients to fully engage in the process, be authentic and vulnerable in a meaningful way, and make progress towards their goals. However, one cannot simply be told, "this is a safe space"; the facilitator is responsible for creating the conditions which allow the participant to feel safe. Creating a psychologically safe space in therapy involves building trust, validating experiences, and fostering a non-judgemental environment where clients feel heard and supported (Newman et al., 2017).

In the context of STP, the LEGO® model and the process of building the model helps to build psychological safety. The participant is given permission to play, and the process itself reinforces that there is no wrong answer. The condition within the permission to play statement (discussed further in Chapter 12) that the model means what the participant tells us it means ensures that assumptions, social norms, or personal values of the facilitator are not imposed on the participant, meaning participants feel free to express themselves without fear of criticism or rejection. The externalisation of thoughts and feelings into the model makes them safe to explore in a non-judgemental and non-threatening way, and because the facilitator can tangibly see what the client is talking about, they feel seen and their perspective understood. Furthermore, any feedback or questions that emerge are directed at the model rather than the builder, increasing the psychological distance and safety for the participant.

Flow theory

The research defines flow as "a state of optimal experience" and an "autotelic experience" (Csíkszentmihályi, 1991). "Autotelic" derives from two Greek words: "autos" (self) and "telos" (end or goal), and the phrase insinuates that such experiences are worth doing in and of themselves. We *feel flow* when we are completely absorbed in a challenging and rewarding activity (and not invested in our inner monologues). People often describe the experience of flow as "being in the zone," a state of concentration so intense that they focus only on the experiences, rather than themselves. In doing so, they lose a sense of time and feel as if there is a merging of their actions and their awareness. During flow, people feel a sense of control and mastery over their skills, allowing them to become more creative and imaginative. In essence, flow experiences are those characterised by immense joy and satisfaction that make life worth living. This understanding inherently aligns with our definitions of play (being intrinsically motivated) and play therapy.

As in play therapy, the experience of flow in STP can be beneficial for clients in several ways. When in flow, clients can develop intrinsic motivation. Flow can help them to develop a sense of self-efficacy, as they become more confident in their abilities to engage in meaningful activities. It can also help them to regulate their emotions, as they become more aware of their feelings and learn how to express them in a healthy way (Jayne & Ray, 2015). Furthermore, the experience of flow itself can be regulated by the client as they choose to build at their own pace, use building techniques that are at their own level of challenge, and titrate their own emotional release.

Relationship

The common third

The concept of *the common third* is typically credited to Michael Husen and has been delineated in two different ways: as a culture and as a process (Pyles & Adam, 2016). As a culture, the common third is about creating a shared situation or context that becomes a symbol of the relationship between the teacher (or, in our case, facilitator) and the student (participant), something "third," or external, to both people that brings them together (Bird & Eichsteller, 2011). In the context of therapy culture, it is, for all intents and purposes, an imaginary space or medium that is created by the interaction between the client and the therapist and which allows for exploration, expression, and growth. Husen (as cited in Pyles & Adam, 2016) suggested that "the common third" can also refer to the shared understanding or interpretation of the context created by the practitioner and the learner.

In an STP approach, the common third moves from an imaginary, intangible sense to a tangible and real object; it has shape, colour, and texture. The LEGO® model becomes the third element in the therapeutic relationship, which can facilitate communication and understanding between the therapist and the client. By focusing on the physical common third produced by the LEGO® and the symbolic meaning imbued in it, the therapist can explore challenges and emotions in a non-threatening way, which can in turn deepen the connection, trust, and collaboration that is essential for effective therapy.

As a process, employing the common third requires finding an activity or context that both the client and the therapist are genuinely interested in and can work together in. In this sense, the common third necessitates a person-centred approach and full participation of the client at every stage, from planning the activity to playing through it to evaluating it afterwards and identifying what has been learned or what has changed (Bird & Eichsteller, 2011). As a result, engaging the common third also eliminates the typical hierarchy seen in therapy, with the therapist as expert and in a position of holding greater procedural knowledge. Equality is created between the client and the therapist as both individuals participate in the activity authentically at the full level of their ability (Hatton, 2020). An equal relationship means that *both* the client and the therapist share a common potential for learning and growth (Bird & Eichsteller, 2011).

STP was conceptualised with the expectation that the practitioner works in an authentic and self-reflective way, bringing their own personality, interests, and strengths, as important resources; this aligns with the intent behind the common third. The benefit of investing in an equal relationship is that the facilitator need not be an expert in LEGO® building. As an individual who has experience with the bricks, you might naturally be a better builder, and as long as the participant has interest in the process, there can be therapeutic value. However, if a participant has more expertise in building, or alternatively, both the facilitator and the participant are novices, there is just as much potential for therapeutic growth.

Like the concepts of psychological safety and flow, the common third is often not a new idea to practitioners. However, by employing these psychological stances with clients, professionals are given language to express the importance of play and logical reasons to argue why STP is valuable in therapeutic contexts. The idea of the common third as context or culture also leads us naturally to the second tenet of our definition of STP: the requirement of relationship.

The present of presence

Bazzano (2013, p. 179) states that "[b]eing present and attentive is the very basic requirement for any practice, of any profession, any work or craft." The concept of *presence* in the craft therapy refers to the therapist's ability to be fully conscious, engaged and attendant in the therapeutic relationship, and to establish a strong connection with the client. It involves being fully attentive to the client, actively listening to them, and creating a safe and supportive environment for them to explore their feelings, thoughts, and experiences (Stadter, 2012). Research suggests that presence has a significant impact on the success of therapy (Grailey et al., 2021). While the concept is fairly straightforward (when the therapist is fully present, the client feels seen, heard, and valued, which can help to build trust and foster a strong therapeutic alliance), the practice is somewhat more challenging to delineate and measure. Within the research, the capacity to investigate is muddied by the understanding of presence on a continuum, with a wholistic, metaphysical experience that cannot be analysed objectively on one end to a quantifiable and measurable experience on the other (Hamilton & Moir-Bussy, 2021). However, qualitative and quantitative explorations cannot accurately account for the complexity of the therapist's presence and its impact in the therapeutic process (Malet et al., 2022). Hamilton and Moir-Bussy (2021) argue that presence exists within spheres or fields, beginning with absence (or a lack of presence) and extending outward in concentric rings to transformative presence, which occurs when both the therapist and the client are able to shift awareness from the self to the potential within the interpersonal interaction.

Achieving the highest levels of presence is highly dependent on the therapist's level of consciousness and involves the therapist being aware of their own thoughts, feelings, and reactions and how these may be influencing the therapeutic relationship. While therapeutic presence is an individual process, STP is understood to support the development of presence through three key factors: mindfulness, active listening, and reflective responses. First, when the therapist engages with the bricks themselves, they are able to be grounded in their own sensation mindful of their own presence. Second, STP facilitates presence by enabling active listening with multiple senses. The therapist pays attention to the client, what they are saying, as well as their body language and tone of voice, but also to the build, what pieces are selected or not, how the model is handled, oriented, or made to be dynamic. Third, reflective responses and questions to the model show their clients that they are being heard and understood. Reflective responses to the model involve acknowledging colours, positions, placements, etc., that the client has shared, which helps the client feel fully seen and heard.

Facilitating communication

As highlighted by Landreth (2012), play is the most natural medium of communication for all children (and, we would argue, for adults as well, as to assume that adults do not benefit from expressing themselves in this natural medium is fundamentally dishonouring to the person; Schaefer, 2003). Play, play therapy, and serious play all facilitate communication by creating a safe and supportive environment where clients can express their understandings, emotions, and experiences. Through play activities, clients can communicate nonverbally, develop language skills, use metaphors to express themselves, and, in the case of therapy, build a strong therapeutic relationship with their therapist (Schaefer & Drewes, 2014).

Even those of us with strong language skills sometimes find it difficult to express our feelings and experiences through words. We discuss in greater detail the role of language in Chapter 5, but what is relevant here is that approaches such as STP do not depend on verbal language and encourage communication through other facets, such as facial expressions, body language, and the play actions used in the building of the model. Through the bricks, the process uses metaphors, storytelling, and storymaking to represent real-life situations and help clients express their emotions and experiences. Children (and adults) may not be able to articulate their thoughts or feelings but they can show them through play and metaphors (Kaduson & Schaefer, 2021). As clients develop their capacity for communication in one medium (in this case, LEGO®), they may be more likely to communicate their thoughts and feelings in other settings and contexts (Schaefer & Drewes, 2014). Furthermore, for those with strongly developed language skills, play-based therapies such as STP can effectively cut through verbal discourse and intellectualisation, often used as a defence in therapeutic approaches (Schaefer, 2003). This allows clients to establish more effective communication patterns and to communicate more directly and authentically.

On the other end of the spectrum, for those with poor language skills or those who have experienced trauma, STP provides an effective, alternative communication medium and gives expression to non-verbalised emotional issues. In essence, the process as well as the bricks themselves provide a language for clients. STP has a unique kinaesthetic quality, which serves the secondary purpose of meeting the client's sensory and kinaesthetic needs and naturally overcoming client resistance and reticence (Kaduson & Schaefer, 2021). The sensory component of working with the LEGO® pieces can promote emotional regulation and self-soothing. This can also bypass neurobiological inhibitions inherent with trauma that limit cognitive processing of verbal language (Sweeney et al., 2014). STP can be particularly helpful for those who may have difficulty expressing themselves through traditional verbalisation.

The common third, the present of presence, and the capacity to facilitate communication are all necessary to the development of an effective therapeutic relationship in an STP approach. However, facilitation of communication may also be a component of the third tenet we initially set forth: intention. The intentions of emotional wellness, learning, and self-reflection are discussed as they relate to STP.

Intention

Emotional wellness

Research continually supports the position that individuals effectively develop emotional awareness and resilience through play, which enables them to manage their emotions, cope with stress, and maintain a positive outlook on life (Schaefer & Drewes, 2014). A strong foundation of emotional wellness can also help children to build positive relationships with others, develop a sense of identity and purpose, and achieve their full potential (Kottman, 2011).

Play and play therapy provide a safe and non-threatening environment for individuals to express their emotions. Once expressed or externalised, play-based interventions provide therapeutic distance. As highlighted in Chapter 3, children play *with* their emotions; they "play" at being scared, excited, angry, and sad. They try out different emotional responses, and in doing so, they learn how to better manage their emotions (Gray, 2019). This therapeutic distance also creates a safe space for abreaction and allows clients to re-experience negative emotions and trauma safely and examine experiences with lowered emotional impact. Play and expressive therapeutic approaches create conditions for clients to experience control and provide boundaries and limits for re-engagement with traumatic or negative experiences, effectively titrating the amount of emotion they experience for themselves. This can be of particular importance with respect to processing traumatic experiences. By re-enacting traumatic events in a safe and controlled environment, individuals can gain a sense of control and mastery over their affective responses (Sweeney et al., 2014).

Within a play therapy context, emotional wellness is a natural focus; the purpose of the engagement in therapy is to support the client in resolving emotional challenges and developing self-regulation, and the therapist has specific training to do so. However, within the context of serious play, while emotions and affective responses can be influenced by various aspects of the game or activity (such as the level of difficulty, the level of collaboration or competition involved, the social dynamics of the group, and the individual's sense of achievement or progress), the purpose of the play is not to explore or resolve these responses. Additionally, the facilitator may or may not have the training or ability to support the participants in emotional regulation. As we have been discussing, STP walks the line between serious play and play therapy. While we make no recommendations about the training or prerequisites required to engage in an STP approach; we would encourage facilitators to consider carefully their capacity and skill in creating and maintaining appropriate conditions to tend to the emotional experience of the participant(s) and to work within their own competency and scope of practice.

Learning

For several years now, there has been a shift in the educational approach from a teaching pedagogy that is based on the "sage on the stage" (King, 1993) to a more constructivist or constructionist approach, where learning is co-created and co-facilitated with the facilitator acting as a "guide on the side" and the participant takes centre stage, actively participating and driving the thinking, creating their own meaning. Play and approaches like STP provide the facilitator and the participant with an excellent environment to step back from the learning and see it afresh (Hamilton, 2019).

Constructivism and constructionism are both based on the idea that knowledge and understanding are constructed by individuals but with slightly different approaches. Constructivism is a theory of learning which posits that knowledge is not simply absorbed and that people must actively construct or make their own knowledge by actively building on the foundation of their current or previous knowledge (Akpan et al., 2020). Social constructivists extend this theory, arguing that learning is a collaborative process and that interaction with others is the central mechanism for knowledge interpretation (Vygotsky, 1978). Vygotsky purported that every function in a child's development occurs twice, "first between people (inter-psychological) and then inside the child (intra-psychological)" (1978, p. 57). By contrast, constructionism is a learning theory hypothesising that learning occurs most effectively when the learner creates, designs, or builds a tangible product that has application in the real world (Papert, 1980). Papert's theory also maintains a social component; both the creation process and the end product must be shared with others to fully construct new knowledge (Papert, 1980; Rob & Rob, 2018). The theories of constructionism and constructivism have many similarities (both begin with an implicit belief in the inherent knowledge of the learner and both are focussed on the development or growth of that learner's knowledge structures) and the terms are often used interchangeably. However, where the two theories are distinguished is in the learning artefact. Constructivism states that the artefact need only be personally meaningful and may or may not be connected to the individual's reality. In constructionism, the artefact must be meaningful within the greater social context and connected to a real-world problem. Furthermore, the artefact must be built through a collaborative creation process (Rob & Rob, 2018).

The rooting of STP in the social constructivist and constructionist theories is clear. The client and counsellor work in relationship to deconstruct maladaptive patterns/behaviours/stories and the counsellor supports the client to rebuild or recreate adaptive ones that facilitate better outcomes (Russo et al., 2006). The link between a constructionist approach and the STP method can be a little more difficult to conceptualise, as it requires two key and counterintuitive competences on the part of the facilitator: first, the facilitator must be willing to work in a more directive manner; and second, they must be willing to invest in the learning artefact of the participant. Working in a directive manner is in opposition to many of the theoretical orientations typically used in play-based approaches, such as Jungian, Person-Centred, or Gestalt (further discussed in Chapter 6). However, while the theoretical orientation guides the therapist in taking on a particular role or stance within the therapeutic relationship, it should not have any bearing on the directive or non-directive nature of the play; this guidance should come from the needs of the child (Yasenik & Gardner, 2012).

The second competence of willingness to invest extends from the collaborative creation process requirement in constructionist approaches. In order for true collaboration to occur, the facilitator must be equally engaged in the creation of the artefact and therefore make effective use of self. In the therapeutic context, use of self refers to how the practitioner draws upon their own feelings, lived experiences, or personality in service of the therapeutic process (Aponte, 2022). However, the research on therapist use of self is mixed; some research suggests that clients are particularly sensitive to counsellors' personal life experiences and perceive responses as more positive and more empathic when the counsellor has made use of some disclosure (Nissen-Lie et al., 2013). Alternatively, Audet (2011) suggests that, when used inappropriately (either in timing or depth), therapist disclosure can diminish perceived credibility and competence.

Self-reflection

In the simplest sense, "self-reflection" refers to the conscious and intentional process of examining one's thoughts, feelings, and behaviours. It involves looking inwardly to gain a deeper understanding of one's motivations, beliefs, and attitudes and to identify patterns of behaviour that may be contributing to current problems, challenges, or stagnation (Seymour & Crenshaw, 2015). In the context of therapy, self-reflection can help clients to explore their emotional reactions and coping mechanisms and gain insight into their interpersonal relationships and the impact of past experiences on their present-day life. However, self-reflective practice is not only for the client. Engagement in the practice on the part of the practitioner is also necessary to do any therapeutic work

(Seymour & Crenshaw, 2015). Most counselling schools or programs require future practitioners to engage in self-reflective practice throughout their training through various modalities (such as the use of learning journals, mindfulness exercises, reviewing videotapes or audio recordings, working with a supervisor, etc.; Young, 2017).

This is yet again another place where STP blurs the line between serious play and play therapy. In serious play, the intent is to solve a particular problem, and the facilitator has promised a solution, whereas no such promise has been made in therapy. The solution to a problem does not inherently require self-reflection. However, as further discussed in Chapter 8, the therapeutic application of a LEGO®-based approach *forces self-reflection*. It is easy to see how this happens for the client: the process of externalising one's thoughts and feelings allows the client to observe them at a safe therapeutic distance and to think objectively about them. However, interestingly, this self-reflection appears to be obligatory for the practitioner as well. When the facilitator works to deepen and expand the client's self-reflection, they must approach the model with non-judgemental curiosity; this requires continuous reflection, to set aside the biases of one's own values, experiences, and feelings and to ask questions with clarity of perspective (Seymour & Crenshaw, 2015).

Conclusion

STP pulls its theoretical grounding from play, play therapy, and serious play. Therapists, facilitators, coaches, and those in the helping professions will recognise that there are no new or previously unknown concepts presented in this chapter. Bringing them together in the context of the psychological state necessary for effective therapeutic intervention, requirements of relationships in an interpersonal process, and intention of the work gives us solid ground from which to work with this new technique.

References

Akpan, V. I., Igwe, U. A., Mpamah, I. B. I., & Okoro, C. O. (2020). Social constructivism: Implications on teaching and learning. *British Journal of Education*, 8(8), 49–56.

Aponte, H. J. (2022). The soul of therapy: The therapist's use of self in the therapeutic relationship. *Contemporary Family Therapy*, *44*, 136–143. https://doi.org/10.1007/s10591-021-09614-5

Audet, C. T. (2011). Client perspectives of therapist self-disclosure: Violating boundaries or removing barriers? *Counselling Psychology Quarterly*, *24*(2), 85–100. https://doi.org/10.1080/09515070.2011.589602

Axline, V. M. (1947). *Play therapy: The inner dynamics of childhood* (L. Carmichael, Ed.). Houghton Mifflin.

Bazzano, M. (2013). Therapeutic presence: A mindful approach to effective therapy by Geller and Greenberg. *Person-Centered & Experiential Psychotherapies*, *12*(2), 177–180. https://doi.org/10.1080/14779757.2013.804653

Bird, V., & Eichsteller, G. (2011). The relevance of social pedagogy in working with young people in residential care. *Good Enough Caring Journal*, *9*. www.goodenough-caring.com/JournalIndex.aspx

Brown, S. (2009). *Play: How it shapes the brain, opens the imagination, and invigorates the soul*. Avery.

Csíkszentmihályi, M. (1991). *Flow: The psychology of optimal experience*. Harper-Perennial.

Frey, D. (2015). Play therapy interventions for adults. In D. A. Crenshaw & A. L. Stewart (Eds.), *Play therapy: A comprehensive guide to theory and practice* (pp. 452–464). The Guilford Press.

Grailey, K. E., Murray, E., Reader, T., & Brett, S. J. (2021). The presence and potential impact of psychological safety in the healthcare setting: An evidence synthesis. *BMC Health Services Research*, *21*(1). https://doi.org/10.1186/s12913-021-06740-6

Grant, A. (2021). *Think again*. Random House UK.

Gray, P. (2019). Evolutionary functions of play: Practice, resilience, innovation, and cooperation. In P. K. Smith & J. Roopnarine (Eds.), *The Cambridge handbook of play: Developmental and disciplinary perspectives* (pp. 84–102). Cambridge University Press. https://doi.org/10.1017/9781108131384.006

Hamilton, A. (2019). *Australian higher education counselling educators' conceptualisation of presence within the context of their teaching* [PhD thesis, University of the Sunshine Coast]. https://doi.org/10.25907/00551

Hamilton, A., & Moir-Bussy, A. (2021). A conceptual analysis of a model of presence within the context of five health professions. *Australian Counselling Research*, *15*(1). www.acrjournal.com.au/resources/assets/journals/Volume-15-Issue-1-2021/Manuscript2%20-%20A%20Conceptual%20Analysis.pdf

Hatton, K. (2020). A new framework for creativity in social pedagogy. *International Journal of Social Pedagogy*, *9*(1). https://doi.org/10.14324/111.444.ijsp.2020.v9.x.016

Jayne, K. M., & Ray, D. C. (2015). Therapist-provided conditions in child-centered play therapy. *The Journal of Humanistic Counseling*, *54*(2), 86–103.

Johnson, S. (2008). *Hold me tight*. Little, Brown Spark.

Kaduson, H. G., & Schaefer, C. E. (Eds.). (2021). *Play therapy with children: Modalities for change*. American Psychological Association.

Kahn, W. A. (1990). Psychological conditions of personal engagement and disengagement at work. *Academy of Management Journal*, *33*(4), 692–724.

Kim, S., Lee, H., & Connerton, T. P. (2020). How psychological safety affects team performance: Mediating role of efficacy and learning behavior. *Frontiers in Psychology*, *11*, 1581–1581. https://doi.org/10.3389/fpsyg.2020.01581

King, A. (1993). From sage on the stage to guide on the side. *College Teaching, 41*(1), 30–35. https://doi.org/10.1080/87567555.1993.9926781

Kottman, T. (2011). *Play therapy: Basics and beyond*. American Counseling Association.

Landreth, G. L. (2012). *Play therapy: The art of the relationship*. Routledge.

Malet, P., Bioy, A., & Santarpia, A. (2022). Clinical perspectives on the notion of presence. *Frontiers in Psychology, 13*. https://doi.org/10.3389/fpsyg.2022.783417

Nachmanovitch, S. (2009). This is play. *New Literary History, 40*(1), 1–24.

Newman, A., Donohue, R., & Eva, N. (2017). Psychological safety: A systematic review of the literature. *Human Resource Management Review, 27*(3), 521–535. https://doi.org/10.1016/j.hmmr.2017.01.001

Nissen-Lie, H. A., Havik, O. E., Høglend, P. A., Monsen, J. T., & Rønnestad, M. H. (2013). The contribution of the quality of therapists' personal lives to the development of the working alliance. *Journal of Counseling Psychology, 60*(4), 483–495. https://doi.org/10.1037/a0033643

Papert, S. A. (1980). *Mindstorms: Children, computers, and powerful ideas*. Basic Books. https://public.ebookcentral.proquest.com/choice/PublicFullRecord.aspx?p=6904793

Pyles, L., & Adam, G. (Eds.). (2016). *Holistic engagement: Transformative education for social workers in the 21st century*. Oxford University Press.

Rob, M., & Rob, F. (2018). Dilemma between constructivism and constructionism. *Journal of International Education in Business, 11*(2), 273–290. https://doi.org/10.1108/JIEB-01-2018-0002

Russo, M. F., Vernam, J., & Wolbert, A. (2006). Sandplay and storytelling: Social constructivism and cognitive development in child counseling. *The Arts in Psychotherapy, 33*(3), 229–237. https://doi.org/10.1016/j.aip.2006.02.005

Schaefer, C. E. (2003). *Play therapy with adults* (pp. xii, 392). John Wiley & Sons.

Schaefer, C. E., & Drewes, A. A. (Eds.). (2014). *The therapeutic powers of play: 20 core agents of change* (2nd ed.). John Wiley & Sons.

Schrage, M. (2000). *Serious play: How the world's best companies stimulate to innovate*. Harvard University Press.

Seymour, J. W., & Crenshaw, D. A. (2015). Reflective practice in play therapy and supervision. In D. A. Crenshaw & A. L. Stewart (Eds.), *Play therapy: A comprehensive guide to theory and practice* (pp. 483–495). The Guilford Press.

Stadter, M. (2012). *Presence and the present: Relationship and time in contemporary psychodynamic therapy*. Jason Aronson.

Statler, M., Heracleous, L., & Jacobs, C. (2011). Serious play as a practice of paradox. *Journal of Applied Behavioural Science, 47*(2), 236–256. https://doi.org/10.1177/0021886311398453

Sweeney, D. S., Baggerly, J., & Ray, D. C. (2014). *Group play therapy: A dynamic approach.* Routledge. https://doi.org/10.4324/9780203103944

United Nations. (1989). *Convention on the rights of the child.* www.ohchr.org/en/instruments-mechanisms/instruments/convention-rights-child

Vygotsky, L. S. (1978). *Mind in society: Development of higher psychological processes* (M. Cole & V. John-Steiner, Eds.). Harvard University Press.

Yasenik, L., & Gardner, K. (2012). *Play therapy dimensions model: A decision-making guide for integrative play therapists* (2nd ed.). Jessica Kingsley Publishers.

Young, M. E. (2017). *Learning the art of helping: Building blocks and techniques* (6th ed.). Pearson.

CHAPTER 5
SPEAKING "LEGO®"
THE PSYCHOLOGY OF LANGUAGE

Kristen Klassen

During the course of my first Master's degree, I was working with children with disabilities, including a number who had a variety of diagnosed learning, language, and communication disorders. Like the inexperienced graduate student I was, I attempted to interview these children as a part of my qualitative research. Of course, this didn't work. It wasn't that the participants in my study didn't have anything to tell me or even that we were not speaking the same language. The children could not verbally express their experience meaningfully and I could not comprehend their message; we were not communicating effectively. As my research progressed, I was introduced to the LEGO® SERIOUS PLAY® method. I integrated pieces of what I had learned in my four-day training into my research model, asking participants to build models of their experience rather than simply having them tell me verbally and my attempts at gathering relevant data and authentic perspectives from my participants were much more successful. The lesson I learnt in this part of my journey was that we all have communication challenges, and we are all collectively responsible for resolving these difficulties.

DOI: 10.4324/9781003260424-6

Limitations of spoken language

My experience working with children with communication disorders is not unique (either to me or to this population). Considerable research from the fields of play and art therapy suggests that verbal language is inherently limiting in the therapeutic relationship (Landreth, 2012; Schaefer & Drewes, 2014; Malchiodi, 2020). First and foremost, the language itself can be a barrier if the therapist and the client do not share a common language. Additionally, language and how we use it is inherently tied to culture, and even if the therapist and client share the same language, they may not share the same cultural context. Cultural differences can impact not only the way that clients express themselves and perceive their experiences but also how they relate to the therapist (Vasquez, 2007).

Although language can be used to represent experience, it also inherently reflects power dynamics and social hierarchies. Bird (2008) has argued that the idea of "correct" or "proper" language use and meaning is often based on arbitrary and subjective rules that reflect the biases and preferences of those in positions of power. Garry Landreth (2012, p. 9) reinforces this position with respect to children, stating that "restricting children to verbal expression automatically places a barrier to a therapeutic relationship by imposing limitations that in effect say to children. 'You must come up to my level and communicate with words.'" Bird (2008) has also pointed out that the notion of linguistic accuracy can be used to marginalise and exclude certain groups of people who speak in ways that are deemed non-standard, or "incorrect." Instead of focusing on notions of correctness or inaccuracy, we should recognise the diversity of language use and appreciate the richness and complexity that comes from this diversity. In the context of therapy, there is clearly a need for greater awareness of the social and cultural context in which a language is used, and for a more inclusive approach to language that recognises and values the contributions of all speakers, regardless of their background or linguistic abilities; STP strives to be this language.

Therapists using an STP approach can overcome many of the limitations presented by reliance on spoken language by using the facets inherent to the STP technique, such as actively "listening" to the model, open-ended questioning and inquiry directed to the model, maintaining and deepening therapeutic metaphors, and prompting of storytelling or storymaking to help clients express themselves fully.

Facilitating communication and actively listening to the model

As discussed in the first three chapters, human brains do not work like a computer; our storage system is much more complex, and the process we utilise to make decisions does not follow a structured, mathematical algorithm. We have multiple sensory inputs for a variety of evolutionary reasons, one of which is to facilitate meaningful communication. Evidence shows that some 40,000 years ago, humans made art that externalised and objectified their experiences. The more permanent nature of the early cave drawings allowed the stories to be seen rather than just heard, allowing them to have a life of their own and to communicate outside the bounds of language and beyond the lifespan of the original artists. To this day, the drawings continue to communicate information (Chakravarthi, 1992).

We introduced the concept of facilitating communication in Chapter 4 as a component of understanding how the STP process depends upon interpersonal relationships as well as enabling emotional expression and regulation. However, the process also facilitates communication by making the unverbalised concepts tangible and concrete and by allowing the facilitator to observe and attend to the intrapsychic and nonverbal components of the interaction.

Nonverbal communication refers to the ways people use body language, gestures, facial expressions, eye contact, tone of voice, proxemics, and other nonverbal cues to convey information and meaning to others. This type of communication can be intentional or unintentional and can heavily influence how a message is received and interpreted (Donovan et al., 2016; Foley & Gentile, 2010). For example, imagine that your partner or a close friend of yours pays you a compliment. Whether they deliver this statement with a relaxed or tense body posture while facing you and making eye contact or looking away, wearing a smile, a frown, or a furrowed brow, with a quick rhythm or a calm cadence and many, many other cues will determine whether you accept the compliment as sincere or reject it as disingenuous. All of these nonverbal cues will also influence how you respond to your partner or friend.

Nonverbal communication is deeply nuanced and depends heavily on cultural, social, and contextual factors (Matsumoto & Hwang, 2016). Taking our compliment example further, imagine the statement was delivered with eye contact. That eye contact might indicate interest, respect, or even aggression, depending on the length and intensity of the gaze. In most Western cultures, eye contact is regarded as positive and is expected, whereas in many others, eye contact is perceived as rude (Foley & Gentile, 2010). For people who are neurodiverse, eye contact can be difficult to make, let alone sustain (Hillary, 2020). Affectively, when people are sad, they tend to make less contact, and when they are happy, they tend to make more (Hills & Lewis, 2011). Yet, therapists are routinely taught to make eye contact themselves and to assess a client's capacity for making and sustaining eye contact (Young, 2017).

In the context of psychotherapy, these nonverbal cues can be further complicated by the client's relationship to not only the therapist but also the process of therapy. Mental health professionals are in a significant position of power over clients by virtue of their education, training, and role (Collins, 2018). Clients who are comfortable with this hierarchy may respond to this power differential with typical nonverbal cues. However, if a client is uncomfortable with this hierarchy, they may present with nonverbal cues of defensiveness or hostility or, alternatively, deference. These nonverbal responses may or may not have any direct connection to the therapeutic conversation taking place. From the therapist's perspective, these nonverbal responses are easily misinterpreted, resulting in missed empathetic opportunities or failure to facilitate perspective taking, ultimately endangering the therapeutic alliance (Vasquez, 2007).

STP strives to hear both the content of the client's words as well as the form. Following the initial request to build a model, the facilitator in the STP context can attend to not only what the participant says about the model but also *how* the participant builds, what pieces they select and what pieces they discard or ignore, the cadence of their building, and other easily distinguishable behaviours. Additionally, eye contact is made to the model, rather than to the person. This transference to the model also reduces reliance on much of the nuanced interpretations of nonverbal behaviours.

Therapeutic metaphor

Metaphors are figures of speech that use a comparison between two things to convey a particular meaning (Lakoff & Johnson, 1980). They are often used to help explain complex ideas or emotions in a way that is more accessible and relatable to the listener. Metaphor is commonly used in therapy as a way to help clients understand and express their emotions and experiences in a way that is both creative and non-threatening

(Gibbs & Matlock, 2008). Davidson (1978) states that "metaphors often make us notice aspects of things we did not notice before; no doubt they bring surprising analogies and similarities to our attention; they provide a kind of lens or lattice, . . . through which we view the relevant phenomena" (p. 45). The benefit of metaphors in a therapeutic context lies in the capacity to create distance from the phenomena; they offer the opportunity to explore difficult emotions and experiences in an indirect manner. This can be especially helpful for clients who have experienced trauma or other forms of adversity, as it can help them to develop coping strategies, capacity for self-regulation, and build emotional resilience (Malchiodi, 2020). Metaphors in therapy can also help clients to develop a sense of control and mastery over their experiences by providing them with a safe and contained space to experience abreaction and to discern alternative outcomes or meanings to difficult experiences (Schaefer & Drewes, 2014).

Part of the power of therapeutic metaphors lies in the psychological processing required to use them. Research in psycholinguistics has shown that the processing of metaphors involves several cognitive processes (Wixted & Thompson-Schill, 2018). First, the listener must recognise the metaphorical nature of the language used. This requires the activation of conceptual knowledge, as the listener must understand the abstract concepts being compared. Once the metaphorical nature of the language is recognised, the listener must then interpret the meaning of the metaphor. This involves mapping the characteristics of the source domain (the concrete or more easily understood concept being used to represent the abstract target domain) onto the target domain (the less concrete or more abstract concept being represented). For example, in the metaphor "Love is a rose," the source domain is the concrete concept of a rose, and the target domain is the abstract concept of love. To interpret this metaphor, the listener must map the characteristics of a rose (e.g., beauty, delicate nature, fragrance, thorns) onto the concept of love. This part of the process relies on context, personal experience, as well as cultural and social conventions. Research has also shown that the processing of metaphors involves different brain regions than the processing of literal language. Specifically, the right hemisphere of the brain, which is associated with the processing of visual and spatial information, appears to be more involved in processing metaphors than the left hemisphere, which is associated with language processing (Ortony, 2018).

As discussed in the biological section of this text, STP engages these cognitive processes by creating more tangible, concrete space with which to overlay the abstract and intangible. This approach is similar to sandtray but with a significant difference; in sandtray, the miniatures and objects used within the tray come imbued with meaning and symbolism (Russo et al., 2006). Therapeutic metaphor is applied to and extends out of the miniatures, resulting in the need for a collection of figures containing "everything that is in the world, everything that has been, everything that can be" (Amatruda & Simpson, 2013, p. 11). In contrast, LEGO® bricks have no inherent meaning, allowing for creative, new, and original metaphors. STP allows the participant the freedom to choose whatever metaphor they can imagine from the bricks; they are not limited to what is available in the prescriptive fashion of miniatures.

However, metaphor is not limited to the spoken word or visual form and exists in other modalities. Metaphor develops naturally in signed languages as well as spoken ones (Meir & Cohen, 2018). Arnheim (1969, p. 118) describes the experience of kinaesthetic metaphor:

> Gestures will act out the pursuit of an argument as though it were a prize fight, showing the weighing of alternatives, the tug of war, the subtle attack, the crushing impact of the victorious retort. This spontaneous use of metaphor demonstrates not only that human beings are naturally aware of the structural resemblance uniting physical and non-physical objects and events; one must go further and assert that the perceptual qualities of shape and motion are present in the very acts of thinking depicted by the gestures and are in fact the medium in which the thinking itself takes place. These perceptual qualities are not necessarily visual or only visual. In gestures, the kinaesthetic experiences of pushing, pulling, advancing, obstructing, are likely to play an important part.

Play and expressive therapies naturally provide the necessary conditions for the emergence of therapeutic metaphors and STP capitalises on this context for building and exploring kinaesthetic metaphors. Kuhn (2022) argues that physical objects (such as LEGO® models) "can also be observed, manipulated, and reconfigured, and by 'talking back', can prompt discovery and cause learners to think in a new way. By moving, juxtaposing, manipulating, and evaluating an object or a combination of objects, new features and opportunities may come to light" (p. 76). The

LEGO® builds participants create in STP provide an opportunity to re-visit their understanding of their experiences, and to test out metaphors in the real world, in real-time. The construction of the model and its associated metaphor(s) provide a refreshed view, a reboot of the senses not only through words and analogies, but through colours, shapes, and movement. The inherent limitations of the bricks create the opportunity for ambiguity, a core feature of metaphor and "a necessary by-product of metaphor's suggestiveness" (Black, 1977, p. 444). This process allows for not only the emergence of kinaesthetic metaphors but also the story-making of potential futures.

Storytelling vs storymaking

Storytelling and storymaking are both ways of engaging with narrative, but there are some important differences between the two. Storytelling involves the act of telling a story that has already been created or writ-ten by someone else. The storyteller uses their voice, tone, and pacing to bring the story to life and engage the listener. Storytelling can be a powerful tool for teaching, entertaining, and transmitting cultural values and traditions. Storymaking, on the other hand, involves the act of creat-ing a story from scratch, often in a collaborative or improvisational way. Storymaking can take many different forms, such as creative writing, role-playing games, or improvisational theatre. The focus is on the cre-ative process of inventing characters, plotlines, and settings, rather than simply retelling an existing story (Smeed, 2012; Buganza et al., 2023).

One of the main differences between storytelling and storymaking is the level of agency and creativity involved. Storytelling involves pre-senting a predetermined narrative to an audience, while storymaking involves actively participating in the creation of a new narrative. Where storytelling is typically understood to be about the past, storymaking is about the future; about the not-yet-known. In storymaking, the par-ticipants have a greater degree of control over the story's direction and outcome (Smeed, 2012; Buganza et al., 2023).

Storymaking and storytelling in application to LEGO® is the basis of an educational program created by LEGO® called StoryStarter. The LEGO® StoryStarter kit includes a range of bricks, minifigures, and a software program that helps students plan, write, and illustrate their sto-ries. Students can use the kit to build scenes and characters and then use the software to capture their creations and turn them into a storyboard.

Although the focus of the program is the development of literacy and language skills through storytelling and storymaking, students also improve their teamwork, problem-solving, abstract reasoning, and critical thinking abilities. The tool encourages creativity and imagination and provides a fun and engaging way for students to learn (LEGO® Education, 2013).

In the context of therapy, both storytelling and storymaking have value in terms of fostering creativity, imagination, and empathy. Storytelling can help to transmit cultural traditions and values, while storymaking can encourage collaborative problem-solving and innovative thinking. While not as prescriptive as the LEGO® StoryStarter approach, STP utilises a similar approach and relies on the same principles. However, rather than curriculum goals with respect to literacy and language development, STP strives to develop social-emotional capacities through the bricks.

The importance of collaborative inquiry to the therapeutic process

Collaborative inquiry is a key aspect of many forms of interpersonal therapy, including narrative therapy, cognitive-behavioural therapy, and solution-focussed therapy (Teyber & Teyber, 2017). In essence, collaborative inquiry involves asking questions that encourage the client to reflect on their experiences, challenge dominant narratives, and develop new ways of thinking about themselves and their lives. Collaborative inquiry can help the client to identify patterns in their thinking and behaviour and to gain insight into the ways in which their past experiences have shaped their current beliefs and attitudes (Taylor de Faoite, 2011).

Collaborative inquiry facilitates therapeutic change by encouraging clients to reflect on their experiences, feelings, and thoughts. Through this process, clients can gain deeper insight into themselves and their situations, which can help them to identify patterns and make connections that they may not have recognised before. Furthermore, clients often come to therapy with dominant narratives about themselves that are negative or limiting. Through collaborative inquiry, therapists can help clients to challenge those narratives and develop new, more empowering stories about themselves and their lives (Taylor de Faoite, 2011). Inquiry prompts clients to consider different perspectives and ways of thinking about their situations. By exploring alternative perspectives, clients can gain a broader understanding of their experiences and develop new ways of thinking and behaving. As clients develop new, more empowering narratives, they can feel more in control of their lives and more capable of making positive changes. By challenging dominant narratives and exploring alternative perspectives, clients can gain a sense of agency and autonomy that can help them to move forward in a positive direction (Morris & Davies, 2018).

The questions we ask in STP (both as prompts to build and in follow-up discussion of built models) are a big part of the therapeutic process. As noted in the introduction, it is *by design* that we do not know what the answer to the question is when we ask it (and, we assume, neither does the client!). Some examples of collaborative inquiry questions that a therapist might use include:

1. What are the dominant stories that you tell yourself about your life?
2. What are some other stories that you could tell about your life that might be more empowering?
3. How have your past experiences influenced your current beliefs and behaviours?

While these types of questions can help the client to develop a more nuanced understanding of their experiences, they are also reliant on linguistic skill (Bird, 2008), limit cognitive processing primarily to the left hemisphere (Ortony, 2018), and do not allow for the emotional distancing necessary for effective processing (Schaefer & Drewes, 2014). In the context of STP, practitioners attempt to ask open-ended questions that allow participants to express themselves freely, without judgement or externally imposed limitations. The previous questions might be modified to include questions like:

1. What's happening in the model right now? Can you show me the movement in the model?
2. How do you feel about what's changed in your build? How might we modify this model to move toward empowerment?
3. Is there anything in your model that defines the current state or past state? I wonder what would happen if you tried something else with the bricks?

These inquiries must still be delivered from a position of non-judge-mental curiosity and with appropriate nonverbal communicators on the part of the facilitator (Tarr, 2021).

Conclusion

By working collaboratively and in a kinaesthetic manner, STP attempts to bypass many of the common limitations to the therapeutic experience presented by reliance on a verbal-language approach. By focusing on the model, the therapist and client work together to explore and understand the client's experiences, thoughts, and feelings in a non-judgemental and supportive way. STP relies on the therapist listening actively to the model and reflecting back on what the client is saying to ensure that they fully understand the client's experience. The therapist and client approach the STP process as equal partners, with the therapist acting as a guide and facilitator rather than an expert or authority figure. STP can be an effective way to promote therapeutic change and help clients to develop new, more empowering narratives that do not rely on language alone.

References

Amatruda, K., & Simpson, P. H. (2013). *Sandplay – the sacred healing: A guide to symbolic process.* Trance*Sand*Dance Press.

Arnheim, R. (1969). *Visual thinking.* University of California Press.

Bird, J. (2008). *Talk that sings: Therapy in a new linguistic key* (2nd ed.). Edge Press.

Black, M. (1977). More about metaphor. *Dialectica, 31*(3–4), 431–457. https://doi.org/10.1111/j.1746-8361.1977.tb01296.x

Buganza, T., Bellis, P., Magnanini, S., Press, J., Shani, A. B., Trabucchi, D., Verganti, R., & Zasa, F. P. (2023). *Storymaking and organizational transformation: How the co-creation of narratives engages people for innovation and transformation.* Routledge. https://doi.org/10.4324/9781003276210

Chakravarthi, P. (1992). The history of communications-from cave drawings to mail messages. *IEEE Aerospace and Electronic Systems Magazine, 7*(4), 30–35. https://doi.org/10.1109/62.143196.

Collins, S. (Ed.). (2018). *Embracing cultural responsivity and social justice: Re-shaping professional identity in counselling psychology.* Counselling Concepts.

Davidson, D. (1978). What metaphors mean. *Critical Inquiry, 5*(1), 31–47. https://doi.org/10.1086/447971

Donovan, J. M., Osborn, K. A. R., & Rice, S. (2016). *Paraverbal communication in psychotherapy: Beyond the words.* Rowman & Littlefield.

Foley, G. N., & Gentile, J. P. (2010). Nonverbal communication in psychotherapy. *Psychiatry, 7*(6), 38–44.

Gibbs, R. W., Jr., & Matlock, T. (2008). Metaphor, imagination, and simulation: Psycholinguistic evidence. In R. W. Gibbs, Jr. (Ed.), *The Cambridge handbook of metaphor and thought* (pp. 161–176). Cambridge University Press. https://doi.org/10.1017/CBO9780511816802.011

Hillary, A. (2020). Neurodiversity and cross-cultural communication. In *Neurodiversity studies* (pp. 91–107). Routledge. https://doi.org/10.4324/9780429322297-10

Hills, P. J., & Lewis, M. B. (2011). Sad people avoid the eyes or happy people focus on the eyes? Mood induction affects facial feature discrimination. *British Journal of Psychology, 102*(2), 260–274. https://doi.org/10.1348/000712610X519314

Kuhn, S. (2022). *Transforming learning through tangible instruction: The case for thinking with things.* Routledge. https://doi.org/10.4324/9781003129073

Lakoff, G., & Johnson, M. (1980). *Metaphors we live by.* The University of Chicago Press.

Landreth, G. L. (2012). *Play therapy: The art of the relationship.* Routledge. https://doi.org/10.4324/9780203835159

LEGO® Education. (2013). Story starter curriculum pack. *Business Wire.* https://le-www-live-s.legocdn.com/downloads/StoryStarter/StoryStarter_Curriculum_1.2_en-GB.pdf

Malchiodi, C. A. (2020). *Trauma and expressive arts therapy: Brain, body, and imagination in the healing process.* Guilford Press.

Matsumoto, D., & Hwang, H. C. (2016). The cultural bases of nonverbal communication. In *APA handbook of nonverbal communication* (pp. 77–101). American Psychological Association. https://doi.org/10.1037/14669-004

Meir, I., & Cohen, A. (2018). Metaphor in sign languages. *Frontiers in Psychology, 9.* https://doi.org/10.3389/fpsyg.2018.01025

Morris, M., & Davies, A. (2018). Being both researcher and subject: Attending to emotion within collaborative inquiry. In *Emotion and the researcher: Sites, subjectivities, and relationships* (Vol. 16, pp. 229–244). Emerald Publishing Limited. https://doi.org/10.1108/S1042-319220180000016015

Ortony, A. (2018). *Some psycholinguistic aspects of metaphor.* Routledge. https://doi.org/10.4324/9780429432866-4

Russo, M. F., Vernam, J., & Wolbert, A. (2006). Sandplay and storytelling: Social constructivism and cognitive development in child counseling. *The Arts in Psychotherapy, 33*(3), 229–237. https://doi.org/10.1016/j.aip.2006.02.005

Schaefer, C. E., & Drewes, A. A. (2014). *The therapeutic powers of play: 20 core agents of change.* John Wiley & Sons.

Smeed, J. (2012). The grumpy dragon and the angry dragon: From storytelling to storymaking. *Storytelling, Self, Society, 8*(1), 1–16.

Tarr, J. (2021). CM 17: Exploring the PACE model – playfulness, acceptance, curiosity, and empathy. *Addressing Issues of Mental Health in Schools through the Arts: Teachers and Music Therapists Working Together, 293.*

Taylor de Faoite, A. (2011). *Narrative play therapy: Theory and practice.* Jessica Kingsley.

Teyber, E., & Teyber, F. H. (2017). *Interpersonal process in therapy: An integrative model* (7th ed.). Cengage Learning.

Vasquez, M. J. T. (2007). Cultural difference and the therapeutic alliance: An evidence-based analysis. *American Psychologist, 62*(8), 878–885. https://doi. org/10.1037/0003-066X.62.8.878

Wixted, J. T., & Thompson-Schill, S. (2018). *Stevens' handbook of experimental psychology and cognitive neuroscience, language and thought: Developmental and social psychology* (4th ed.). John Wiley & Sons. https://doi.org/10.1002/9781119170174

Young, M. E. (2017). *Learning the art of helping: Building blocks and techniques* (6th ed.). Pearson.

CHAPTER 6
BREAKING DOWN BRICK WALLS
THE RELATIONSHIP OF STP TO THE THERAPEUTIC DISCIPLINES

Kristen Klassen

The importance of approaching any therapeutic intervention from sound theoretical ground cannot be overstated; the clinical approach from which one operates orients a clinician's view of the client, the experiences and challenges of their client, and their understanding and view of the world. In essence, clinical theory provides the treatment planning road map for the therapeutic journey and the compass for guidance.

Therapists are commonly asked about their theoretical orientation, to which the answer for many modern practitioners is "eclectic" or "integrative." Using multiple theoretical groundings in and of itself is not problematic and has spawned a new approach to research and clinical work based on the "common factors" between theoretical orientations (Wampold, 2015). What has resulted is a generation of practitioners who, while less dogmatic in their approach, are also less invested or anchored in any one theoretical approach to assessment and treatment (Bailey & Ogles, 2019). This, in turn, may be problematic, as a therapist will interact differently with a client based on their own beliefs. For example, the interventions a clinician might use if they believe that a client is innately creative and therefore capable of self-actualizing (such as in a person-centred orientation) would be quite different from those they might use if they believe that a client must be taught how to recognise

DOI: 10.4324/9781003260424-7

and correct irrational or distorted thinking (as in a cognitive-behavioural understanding).

A full exploration of the various theories is beyond the scope of this book; in many cases, examining the assorted theoretical orientations is a full course or multiple courses as a part of a graduate training program. However, returning to our initial tenet, practitioners need a sound theoretical orientation to enact therapeutic change. Fall et al. (2017, p. 9) argue that your theoretical approach is already embedded within you; "you already have beliefs about what causes people to be as they are and what they need to continue in their development; in the process of living, you have already begun to develop your own fledgling guidebook." Therefore, this section aims to align STP with the beliefs that underlie the more commonly used theoretical orientations.

We present STP as a modality; it is a communication and expression process rather than a codified method or theory of psychotherapy in and of itself. This means that, similar to approaches such as sandplay or art therapy, the technique can be useful in many theoretical toolboxes (or "tickle trunks," as the case may be!). We hope you can integrate STP no matter which theoretical orientation you utilise in your therapeutic approach to clients. We will now explore the relationship between STP and some major theoretical orientations, again remembering that this is not intended to be exhaustive (or fully descriptive) of the theories presented. We conclude by discussing STP's value and limitations as an assessment technique.

Psychoanalytic/analytical psychology orientations

Psychoanalytic theory, traditionally attributed to the work of Freud, is less of a unified theory of personality or treatment and more of a collection of basic principles. Foremost among these is the assertion that humans are motivated by fantasies, wishes, dreams, or other tacit knowledge outside of awareness. Knowing that people work to avoid painful or threatening fantasies or memories, a primary goal in psychoanalytic therapy is to facilitate awareness of one's unconscious motivations, thus allowing one to make more reasoned and productive decisions (Safran et al., 2019).

STP fits within psychoanalytic theory, as it also works to uncover the unconscious; the primary goal in using LEGO® bricks is to access the estimated 95% of cognitive activity that we are not consciously aware of

(Kastrup, 2017). Embodiment processes are those practices that make manifest or comprehensible an idea or concept through a physical presentation. Utilising the inherent and necessary interconnections between body and mind (Kuhn, 2022), STP seeks to reunite the processes of cognition and perception through the physical medium and bring the unconscious mind to consciousness. Psychoanalytic inquiry skills can then be used to deepen the understanding of what has emerged from the unconscious. The skill of the therapist or facilitator in an STP approach is to guide the participant to those places where further exploration may be of value.

Another core principle within psychoanalytic approaches is the use and understanding of transference (and countertransference), the act of projecting feelings or experiences to another person or object (or outward expression). Freud's understanding of transference was that it was indispensable to understanding how past experiences influenced the present emotional state (Freud, 1958). However, transference requires therapists to be able to tolerate and process painful and disturbing emotions (both from the client and within themselves) in a non-judgmental way (Ekman & Davidson, 1994). STP intentionally makes use of this principle to assist the client to project their transference onto a LEGO® build, aiming to help them experience a level of containment for the emotional content. Having the feelings projected externally to both the therapist and the client allows the therapist to focus on helping the client process and regulate their emotions (as opposed to regulating their own emotional experience).

Finally, within psychoanalytic approaches, it is understood that the therapeutic relationship is the primary vehicle for change. Psychoanalytic practitioners believe it is inevitable that they will fail the client by not being attuned to their needs, resulting in the client re-experiencing their trauma. However, the therapist's failure is viewed as an opportunity to work through the initial trauma in a constructive fashion and repair the therapeutic relationship (Fall et al., 2017). Again, STP works productively to allow the client and therapist to rebuild and reconstruct their relationship as frequently – and as differently – as necessary.

Carl Jung, a colleague of Freud, was originally a follower of the school of psychoanalysis. He ultimately disagreed with Freud's framework and founded his own school of thought (Analytical Psychology). Jung posited that the human psyche consists of the ego, the personal unconscious, and the collective unconscious. Jung's concept of the ego (the conscious mind that contains the awareness of existing and the sense of personal identity) was similar, in many ways, to Freud's formulation of the ego. However, Jung's understanding of the unconscious is where the theories diverged. Jung theorised that the personal unconscious is composed of memories that are subliminal, forgotten, or repressed, whereas the collective unconscious (or transpersonal unconscious) is a universal experience of the personal unconscious, shared with all members of the human species. These shared ancestral memories, born from evolution, are called archetypes and are represented by universal themes that appear in various cultures. Each archetype is two-sided, having both positive and negative poles, and Jungian therapists suggest that, when problems arise, they are due to an archetypal imbalance (Schultz & Schultz, 2017).

Like Jungian approaches to other three-dimensional techniques, such as sandplay (Roesler, 2019), STP can be used effectively from a Jungian orientation. The therapist invites the client to build a model with LEGO®. As the client builds, their psyche concurrently explores and re-evaluates the new and potentially healthier configurations developed through the build. This takes place with no intermediary, as the building hands link directly with the psyche, developing the physical, three-dimensional model that allows the "modelling" and "remodelling" of the mental configuration towards a healthier, fuller functioning. Furthermore, the modelling takes place in our first and most natural language of symbolism and therefore bypasses the intricacies and limitations of spoken communication.

Individuation is "the gradual development of a unified, integrated personality that incorporates greater and greater amounts of the unconscious, both personal and collective, and resolves any conflicts that exist, such as those between introverted and extraverted tendencies" (American Psychological Association, 2015). Jung believed that, for individuation to occur, the personal unconscious and the conscious ego must be fully integrated. In essence, the therapeutic goal of individuation within analytic psychology is the process through which a person becomes a whole psychological individual. The individual works towards recognising their self-worth and uniqueness and embraces both their conscious and unconscious selves (Schultz & Schultz, 2017).

Recognition of one's own self-worth and uniqueness is a natural objective of the STP process; in the introduction to the technique in therapy, the client (builder) is reminded that there is no wrong answer to the question(s). The purpose of this approach is to help the client hear their own unique perspective in their own voice, see their own unique viewpoint in 3-D, and find value in that perspective.

Cognitive-Behavioural Therapy (CBT) and Rational Emotive Behavioural Therapy (REBT)

Cognitive Behavioural Therapy (CBT) is rooted in the cognitive approach presented by Aaron Beck. CBT differs from many other therapeutic approaches because it focuses on helping individuals learn to identify the relationship between their thoughts, feelings, and behaviours. While each of these are interdependent (they all serve to influence each other), CBT gives special attention to the role of cognition (automatic thoughts, rules and assumptions, and core beliefs) in creating and maintaining emotional difficulties such as depression and anxiety. CBT aims to help clients identify, evaluate, and change their habitual thinking patterns at each of these levels of cognition. Working with the therapist, one learns that assigning less extreme, more helpful, and more accurate meanings to negative events leads to less extreme and disturbing emotional and behavioural responses. Once clients have learnt these skills in therapy, they become their own therapists, able to manage difficult experiences and emotional upset on their own (Kennerley et al., 2017).

A unique feature of CBT approaches is the distinction between a therapeutic relationship and a therapeutic alliance; while most therapeutic methodologies focus on an alliance resulting from alignment goals and tasks in the therapeutic intervention, CBT focuses on the exchange of thoughts and feelings to facilitate meaningful change for the client (Okamoto et al., 2019). This differentiation means that the therapist can disagree with the underlying core beliefs of the client but still be empathetic and genuine in working with the client (Beck & Weishar, 2019). However, as Kennerley et al. (2017) cautioned, the therapist must be aware of the frames of reference within which they operate and evaluate their own core beliefs to avoid violating the non-judgement principle of the CBT approach. CBT is understood to translate well to various belief systems, provided the therapist acknowledges their perspective and blind spots and shows respect for the client's culture.

Rational Emotive Behaviour Therapy was developed by clinical psychologist Albert Ellis and works on the premise that one's perceptions of events lead to emotional, behavioural, and relational challenges. Ellis and Ellis (2019) argued that humans are born with the potential to be rational and constructive as well as irrational and destructive. Where CBT therapists focus primarily on cognitive distortions, REBT practitioners focus on irrational beliefs and thoughts held by the client.

There is a natural connection between STP and CBT/REBT approaches in that the medium of LEGO® helps the client to develop an awareness of their thoughts and feelings as they build and work to make them tangible. Furthermore, STP questions can intentionally address cognitive distortions and irrational beliefs. In contrast to other approaches, REBT and CBT therapists do not rely on the therapeutic relationship. With respect to STP, this may help reduce any external judgement the client may experience within the therapeutic journey. It is not essential for the therapist to like the model, but rather, to understand it from the client's perspective and assist the client in deepening their understanding of it.

Person-centred

Originally formulated by Carl Rogers, "Person-Centred" theory assumes that people can achieve self-understanding and self-actualisation when they experience a relationship with a therapist who is genuine, congruent, and offers unconditional positive regard for them (Raskin et al., 2019). Person-centred or client-centred approaches differ from other interventions in their commitment to a non-directive attitude; the therapist strives to respect the client and their worldview and validate and accept whatever the client chooses to share.

The work of Rogers was extended into the realm of play therapy by Virginia Axline (1947), who operationalised the principles and theories of person-centred therapy to relationships with children. Child-Centered Play Therapy (CCPT) is now the most used theoretical orientation with the strongest research base (Landreth, 2012). Axline's approach is based on the belief that all children's behaviour and outward expression result from the drive for self-actualisation. The child-centered play therapist creates a space where the child is free to play with toys and materials of their choosing, without any pressure or direction from the therapist (Axline, 1947). The therapist observes the child's play and offers empathy, validation, and support, as needed, but does not direct the child's play or offer solutions to problems, and in doing so, enables the child to achieve self-awareness and self-direction (Landreth, 2012).

From this perspective, person-centred approaches are a natural fit with STP. Rogers famously asked, "So I have learned to ask myself, can I hear the sounds and sense the shape of this other person's inner world?" (Rogers, 1995, p. 8). The LEGO® build the client creates allows the facilitator to not only hear the sounds of the client's inner world as they tell their story in their own words but to observe the shapes and colours as they are made tangible. The facilitator may even bear witness to the client's perspective interactively as the metaphor is acted out. The facilitator does not analyse the client, nor give explicit advice or guidance to the client. Instead, the facilitator takes an active role in the session by observing the client's build, listening closely to the client's story, asking questions to the model, and helping the client to gain insight into their own experiences through the model.

Gestalt

Gestalt therapy is primarily attributed to the work of Fritz Perls and his two collaborators, Laura Perls and Paul Goodman. The word "gestalt" comes from the German word for "whole," and in therapy, it refers to the idea that people have a natural tendency to perceive their experiences as unified "wholes" rather than separate parts (Milić, 2020). The interventions used are experiential in nature and based on the idea that people are naturally creative and have the capacity to change themselves and their situations. The therapist's role is to help clients become more aware of their thoughts, feelings, and behaviours and to support them in taking responsibility for their own lives (Yontef & Jacobs, 2019).

In contrast to the previous orientations discussed, Gestalt therapy focuses on a person's present life and current challenges rather than on past experiences that many other therapies delve into (Mann, 2010). Clients are encouraged to focus on their immediate experiences and to become more aware of their bodily sensations, emotions, and thoughts. Through this process, the therapist guides them to gain insight into their patterns of behaviour and develop new ways of responding to their environment (Yontef & Jacobs, 2019). STP and the use of physical or tangible tools such as LEGO® are valuable assets in maintaining awareness of the present. As Kuhn (2022) highlights, tangible objects can help clients ground themselves in the present moment and feel more connected to their physical bodies. The LEGO® pieces can also be used as sensory stimulation (feeling the edges of the pieces, the lightness, or smoothness, seeing the vibrancy of the colours, etc.), facilitating the practice of affect labelling (accurately and precisely naming a sensation or emotion), and supporting the client in fully experiencing the present moment. Paul (2022) further suggests that accurately distinguishing interoceptive sensations is associated with reducing psychological arousal, allowing for better decision-making and less impulsive actions.

Another key aspect of gestalt therapy is the use of experiential techniques (such as role-playing, empty-chair work, and creative expression) designed to help clients explore and express their emotions and experiences in a more direct and immediate way (Mann, 2010; Neukrug, 2015). Gestalt therapy utilises three foundational pillars in experiential treatments: *field* refers to the interaction between an individual and their environment, *dialogue* refers to the here-and-now conversation, and *phenomenology* refers to the authentic experience of the phenomenon by the individual (Milić, 2020). With an effective therapist, the therapeutic technique of STP engages all three pillars; the LEGO® build is both a conduit between the individual and their environment and an artefact of the phenomenological experience of the client. The build also becomes the basis for the here-and-now dialogue and an anchor point, should the client venture into the past or future. The ultimate goal of the STP technique within a Gestalt approach is to restore the client's self-regulation and sense of self (Yontef & Jacobs, 2019).

Narrative

Narrative therapy is rooted in the social constructivist approach and belief that each individual is the expert in their own life, with many skills, competencies, values, commitments, and abilities to support them. As an approach, it seeks to be respectful and non-blaming and views problems as separate from people. As a therapeutic orientation, it emerged in the 1980s from the work of David Epston and Michael White (White, 2007).

A key tenet of narrative interventions is externalisation; putting together the story of their lives allows people to observe themselves and their challenges separate from their being. This helps create distance between the individual and their problems and allows people to focus better on changing unwanted behaviours. As people practise externalisation, they get the opportunity to see that they are capable and empowered to change (White, 2007). STP can be approached as a means of externalisation; one can physically view the story they have built as external to themselves. The process allows individuals to work through challenging emotions, thoughts, and feelings without having to identify and label them or claim them as a part of themselves. The LEGO® model, in essence, provides distancing from and containment for the actual experience(s) or event(s), enabling individuals to deal with an intense emotional response without being overwhelmed by the experience itself.

When a story feels cemented in a person's life and they feel things can never change, any idea of alternative stories seems impossible. People can become very stuck in their stories, negatively influencing areas of their lives and impacting decision-making, behaviours, experiences, and relationships. A narrative therapist works to help people not only challenge their problems but widen their views by considering alternative stories (Marsten et al., 2016). The process of building in STP facilitates this challenging process by assisting the facilitator in wondering out loud about the model and its structure, "How this might be helpful in telling a new story today?" or "How might the model be built differently now that you know XYZ?".

The process of deconstruction is also used to help people gain clarity in their stories. When a problematic story feels like it has been around for a long time, people might use generalised statements, become confused, or fixed in their stories. A narrative therapist works with the individual to break down the story into smaller parts, clarifying the problem and making it more approachable (Freeman et al., 1997). Deconstructing the LEGO® build of a problematic story facilitates this process, where the client can physically pull apart various aspects of their story that are no longer useful or helpful.

Solution-focussed

Solution-focussed brief therapy (SFBT) was developed in the early 1980s by Insoo Kim Berg and Steve de Shazer and uses a goal-directed approach to find solutions to problems. This orientation is also based in constructivist approaches and is future-focussed, prioritising discovering current resources and strengths that will facilitate solutions instead of focusing on the past or the problem. In contrast to many other orientations, the approach was formed deductively; Berg and Shazer spent hundreds of hours, across many years, observing therapy sessions and methodically noted the questions, behaviours, and emotions that led clients to real-life solutions. Based on this data, the SFBT approach incorporated only the questions that consistently demonstrated client progress and solutions. Meanwhile, questions or statements that did not provide real growth or problem-solving were eliminated (Ratner et al., 2012).

In alignment with STP, SFBT practitioners are trained to approach each case non-judgementally. Clients are empowered to make their own goals rather than relying on the therapist to lead the way. This therapy approach allows clients to identify the problem-solving skills they need to improve their self-esteem and forward-thinking. As discussed, many traditional therapeutic orientations revolve around past life-events and problems to uncover deeper significance, whereas SFBT motivates clients to focus on the present to achieve future goals. This approach is built around optimism and positivity psychology. It identifies steps that can be taken today to improve the client's day tomorrow (or the immediate short-term) (Neukrug, 2015). The STP facilitator, under this approach, would prompt the client to build towards the future or build a situation where the problem is not present. This build might then be examined with a view of "How do we get there?" or "What aspect of the build helps you find yourself in solution rather than problem?".

Common factors

Common factors therapeutic orientation is a modern approach to therapy that focuses on identifying and utilising the common elements that are effective across different types of therapies, rather than adhering to one specific theoretical approach. This approach purports that, while specific interventions may target specific psychological problems (i.e., CBT for anxiety), the evidence indicates that the individual components derived from specific theoretical approaches account for minimal differences in the outcome variance when measuring treatment effectiveness. Furthermore, the commonly occurring elements in all methods (such as the client's experience of the relationship, the creation of hope and setting of expectations, and the qualities of the therapist) are responsible for a much larger proportion of outcome variance (Neukrug, 2015).

Researchers disagree on which factors are critical to successful therapy (Cuijpers et al., 2019; Tschacher et al., 2014); however, some consistent factors that emerge are: (1) a strong therapeutic alliance between the therapist and the client, built on trust, mutual respect, and open communication; (2) a non-judgemental environment in which the client feels safe to explore their feelings and concerns; (3) the instillation of hope and a motivation to achieve change for the client; (4) active listening and empathy on the part of the therapist, who recognises the importance of understanding the client's unique perspective, experiences, and needs and validates the client's feelings; and (5) therapy is viewed as a collaborative process, with the therapist and client working together to identify goals, develop strategies, and monitor progress (Neukrug, 2015).

Overall, the common factors therapeutic orientation emphasises the importance of individualising treatment to the client and utilising a flexible approach that draws from a variety of therapeutic techniques and theories (Neukrug, 2015). Again, this aligns with an STP intervention; as highlighted throughout this section, the technique can be successfully adapted to the majority of philosophical understandings of the therapeutic process, and a common factors approach is no different.

Using STP in assessment

Research suggests that play therapy can be a useful tool for assessment, particularly for individuals who may have difficulty expressing their thoughts and feelings through traditional talk therapy methods or may not have fluency in the same language as the therapist. In a play therapy assessment, a therapist observes a child playing with toys or engaging in other creative activities, such as drawing or storytelling. The therapist may also join in the play to help build rapport and create a safe and supportive environment. Through this observation and interaction, the therapist can gain insight into the child's emotional state, behaviours, and thought patterns, allowing them to develop an appropriate treatment plan (Chazan, 2002).

Play therapy and similar approaches can be particularly effective for assessing social skills, communication skills, emotional regulation, and cognitive development. For example, a therapist may observe how a child interacts with peers or caregivers during play, or how they express emotions such as anger or sadness. The therapist may also note how the child problem-solves or copes with challenges presented during play (Chazan, 2002; Kottman, 2011). However, there are some limits to the use of play in psychological assessment. First, play behaviour is not always a reliable indicator, as it can be influenced by many factors (such as the client's mood, level of comfort, and the presence of others in the room), meaning that the client may behave differently during different play sessions or play activities. This can make it difficult to draw accurate conclusions about personality, behavioural challenges, or emotional state.

Additionally, play assessments can be time-consuming and require specialised training to administer and interpret. This can make it difficult for clinicians or researchers to use play assessments on a large scale or in settings where resources are limited. Furthermore, some researchers and clinicians have questioned the validity of play assessments, arguing that they rely heavily on subjective interpretations of play behaviour rather than standardised measures (Schaefer et al., 2005; O'Connor & Ammen, 2013).

We cannot stress enough that STP is process driven and is not intended to be the base for analysis out of context. STP should not be used as the sole method of assessment but should be used in conjunction with other assessment tools, such as interviews, questionnaires, standardised assessments, and any other measures included in the therapist's training or scope of practice. If STP is used as part of an assessment, a trained therapist should conduct the assessment to ensure the results are accurate and meaningful. While play can be a valuable tool for psychological assessment in certain situations, it should not be relied on exclusively, and STP is no different.

Conclusion

My personal theoretical orientation is rooted in the humanistic and constructivist approaches, and in my playroom, I operate primarily from a non-directive approach (and I gather from our conversations that my co-authors work in similar ways). I believe that the primary benefit of STP lies in the intrapsychic and interpersonal safety that is inherent in the technique. However, writing this chapter and thinking through how STP might be conceptualised within those approaches I do not employ was an exercise in understanding the potential of this new tool and how the technique might be adapted to fit within more structured orientations.

As noted in the introduction, this chapter is not a comprehensive review of all of the possible theoretical approaches. We hope that we have highlighted for you the most commonly used approaches and that you have found some alignment and understanding of how the STP process might fit within your own understanding and approach to delivering therapeutic interventions. Your theoretical orientation supports you in understanding your client and their presentation and guides your clinical decision-making, intervention selection, and treatment planning; we hope we have made a strong argument for including STP in your approach.

References

American Psychological Association. (2015). *APA dictionary of psychology*. American Psychological Association.

Axline, V. M. (1947). *Play therapy: The inner dynamics of childhood* (L. Carmichael, Ed.). Houghton Mifflin.

Bailey, R. J., & Ogles, B. M. (2019). Common factors as a therapeutic approach: What is required? *Practice Innovations*, 4(4), 241–254. https://doi.org/10.1037/pri0000100

Beck, A. T., & Weishar, M. E. (2019). Cognitive therapy. In D. Wedding & R. J. Corsini (Eds.), *Current psychotherapies* (11th ed., pp. 237–272). Cengage Learning.

Chazan, S. E. (2002). *Profiles of play: Assessing and observing structure and process in play therapy*. J. Kingsley.

Cuijpers, P., Reijnders, M., & Huibers, M. J. H. (2019). The role of common factors in psychotherapy outcomes. *Annual Review of Clinical Psychology*, 15, 207–231. https://doi.org/10.1146/annurev-clinpsy-050718-095424

Ekman, P., & Davidson, R. J. E. (1994). *The nature of emotions: Fundamental questions*. Oxford University Press.

Ellis, A., & Ellis, D. J. (2019). Rational emotive behaviour therapy. In D. Wedding & R. J. Corsini (Eds.), *Current psychotherapies* (11th ed., pp. 157–198). Cengage Learning. https://doi.org/10.1037/0000134-000

Fall, K., Miner Holden, J., & Marquis, A. (2017). *Theoretical models of counseling and psychotherapy* (3rd ed.). Routledge. https://doi.org/10.4324/9781315733531

Freeman, J., Epston, D., & Lobovits, D. (1997). *Playful approaches to serious problems: Narrative therapy with children and their families*. W. W. Norton & Company.

Freud, S. (1958). *The dynamics of transference* (Standard, Vol. 12). Hogarth Press.

Kastrup, B. (2017). There is an "unconscious," but it may as well be conscious. *Europe's Journal of Psychology*, 13(3), 559–572. https://doi.org/10.5964/ejop.v13i3.1388

Kennerley, H., Kirk, J., & Westbrook, D. (2017). *An introduction to cognitive behaviour therapy – skills and applications* (3rd ed.). SAGE Publications.

Kottman, T. (2011). *Play therapy: The basics and beyond* (2nd ed.). American Counseling Association.

Kuhn, S. (2022). *Transforming learning through tangible instruction: The case for thinking with things*. Routledge. https://doi.org/10.4324/9781003129073

Landreth, G. L. (2012). *Play therapy: The art of the relationship*. Routledge. https://doi.org/10.4324/9780203835159

Mann, D. (2010). *Gestalt therapy: 100 key points and techniques*. Routledge.

Marsten, D., Epston, D., & Markham, L. (2016). *Narrative therapy in wonderland: Connecting with children's imaginative know-how*. W. W. Norton & Company.

Milić, J. (2020). Gestalt psychotherapy: Science or quasi-science? *Acta Medica Medianae*, 59(1), 158. https://doi.org/10.5633/amm.2020.0124

Neukrug, E. S. (Ed.). (2015). *The SAGE encyclopedia of theory in counseling and psychotherapy*. SAGE Publications. https://doi.org/10.4135/9781483346502

O'Connor, K. J., & Ammen, S. (2013). *Play therapy treatment planning and interventions: The ecosystemic model and workbook* (2nd ed.). Elselvier. https://doidoi.org/10.1016/B978-0-12-373652-9.00007-8.

Okamoto, A., Dattilio, F. M., Dobson, K. S., & Kazantzis, N. (2019). The therapeutic relationship in cognitive-behavioral therapy: Essential features and common challenges. *Practice Innovations*, *4*(2), 112–123. https://doi.org/10.1037/pri0000088

Paul, A. M. (2022). *The extended mind: The power of thinking outside the brain.* Mariner.

Raskin, N. J., Rogers, C. R., & Witty, M. C. (2019). Client-centered therapy. In D. Wedding & R. J. Corsini (Eds.), *Current psychotherapies* (11th ed., pp. 101–156). Cengage Learning.

Ratner, H., George, E., & Iveson, C. (2012). *Solution focused brief therapy: 100 key points and techniques (Ser. 100 key points)*. Routledge.

Roesler, C. (2019). Sandplay therapy: An overview of theory, applications and evidence base. *The Arts in Psychotherapy*, *64*, 84–94. https://doi.org/10.1016/j.aip.2019.04.001

Rogers, C. R. (1995). *A way of being.* Houghton Mifflin.

Safran, J. D., Kriss, A., & Foley, V. K. (2019). Psychodynamic psychotherapies. In D. Wedding & R. J. Corsini (Eds.), *Current psychotherapies* (11th ed., pp. 21–57). Cengage Learning.

Schaefer, C., McCormick, J., & Ohnogi, A. J. (2005). *International handbook of play therapy: Advances in assessment, theory, research, and practice.* Jason Aronson.

Schultz, D. P., & Schultz, S. E. (2017). *Theories of personality* (11th ed.). Cengage Learning.

Tschacher, W., Junghan, U. M., & Pfammatter, M. (2014). Towards a taxonomy of common factors in psychotherapy-results of an expert survey. *Clinical Psychology & Psychotherapy*, *21*(1), 82–96. https://doi.org/10.1002/cpp.1822

Wampold, B. E. (2015). How important are the common factors in psychotherapy? An update. *World Psychiatry*, *14*(3), 270–277. https://doi.org/10.1002/wps.20238

White, M. (2007). *Maps of narrative practice.* W. W. Norton & Company.

Yontef, G., & Jacobs, L. (2019). Gestalt therapy. In D. Wedding & R. J. Corsini (Eds.), *Current psychotherapies* (11th ed., pp. 309–348). Cengage Learning.

CHAPTER 7
THE SOCIAL SIDE OF HEALTH
BUILDING RELATIONSHIPS

Mary Anne Peabody

As the overall framework of this book, we have embraced the biopsychosocial model as an integrated and holistic approach. For years, the biopsychosocial model has permeated the rhetoric of health psychology, as this model of care offers a client-centred approach where all three factors – social, psychological and biological – are considered alongside each other. Each of the three factors is characteristically different, but none functions independently.

Therefore, this chapter extends the biopsychosocial model by adding another layer of conceptual thinking to include human ecologies. According to (Berns, 2016, p. 5), ecology is the science of interrelationships between organisms and their environments. Therefore, human ecology includes the biological, psychological, social, and cultural contexts in which a person interacts with various environments over time (Bronfenbrenner & Morris, 2006). One important feature of an ecological systems approach is the assumption that all factors within and across the systems are "interrelated and mutually influential," from the level of the individual through groups to the macro-level of society (Moran et al., 2016, p. 135). This interactional interdependence between and within different parts of the environment or ecologies dynamically occurs across the life span. How these parts reciprocally affect and are affected by one

DOI: 10.4324/9781003260424-8

another are critical drivers of treatment progression that, in turn, impact how individuals cope and behave.

The developmental psychologist Urie Bronfenbrenner (1979) stands out as one of the most influential contributors to ecological thinking in health research. Bronfenbrenner's (1979, 1995, 2005) ecological systems theory maintains that human development is profoundly influenced by a nested set of systems ranging from the intimate to those systems more removed from the individual (Bronfenbrenner, 1979). Changes in any of these systems affect the smaller systems that reside within them and, ultimately, the developmental pathway of the individual. The following quote from (Bronfenbrenner, 2005) speaks to the ever-changing social nature of human development.

> Human beings create environments that shape the course of human development. Their actions influence the multiple physical and cultural tiers of the ecology that shapes them, and this agency makes humans – for better or worse – active producers of their own development.
>
> (p. xxvii)

According to Bronfenbrenner's ecological theory (1995), there are five basic structural systems: 1) the microsystem, 2) the mesosystem, 3) the exosystem, and 4) the macrosystem. These four systems are influenced by broader social change in the fifth system: 5) the chronosystem that includes economics, technology, and politics. As you read the system examples put forth by Berns (2016), you discover some level of overlapping between the ecologies; however, for our purposes, the individual's interactions with and between systems are the focus.

Berns provides descriptions and examples of ecologies:

- The microsystem refers to relationships with significant others, typically including family, school, neighbourhood, peer group, community, and media.
- The mesosystem consists of linkages and interrelationships between two or more microsystems; for example, family and school, family and clubs, or interactional professional or personal networks.
- The exosystem is the structure where the individual is not an active participant; however, the system affects them. For example,

a parent's working hours impact a child's development; a parent's employment impacts family members' type, level, or access to health insurance benefits. An adult example could be decisions that a city council planning board makes on whether a park or a high-rise apartment building will be constructed in a specific area and the impact on green space or property values.

- The macrosystem is the larger society comprised of a community, nation, or a broad group of individuals that possess common traditions, activities, or interests. With macrosystems, subcultures can form and impact an individual's lifestyle, social interactions, and belief systems. For example, religious groups; urban vs. rural living and values; political ideology, science and technology access, and beliefs.

- The chronosystem: the interaction of the ecological systems over time. The COVID pandemic is a chronosystem example, impacting all individuals temporally and across numerous ecologies. Other chronosystem system changes that have changed over time include: changes in airport security due to terrorist attacks; information technology access through internet, cell-phone, and artificial intelligence access. Naturally, depending on access and environment these changes may vary in how the human experience is altered.

Lastly, the application of systems theory to the study of health acknowledges the contextual nature of relationships and recognises that interpersonal relationships exist in symbiosis with wider relationships nested within school, work, community, and public or human services. This relational approach demands a conceptual shift from thinking only about individuals to a more holistic paradigm, or a more "socially embodied individual" – located in the context of their interrelationships and social practices that make up their everyday experiences.

The social side of health

Psychologists, sociologists, and epidemiologists have contributed greatly to our understanding of how social processes influence physiological processes. This understanding helps explain the linkages between social ties, social support, and health across the lifespan. Throughout development, humans are exposed to social conditions that promote or undermine health, and over time, these exposures accumulate to create growing health advantages or disadvantages in socially patterned ways.

These social conditions shape health behaviour because they influence and shape our health habits (Umberson et al., 2010). For example, social ties can instil a sense of responsibility and concern for others, leading individuals to engage in positive behaviours that protect their own health as well as the health of others. Alternatively, social ties can influence negative choices or behaviours, leading to unhealthy actions. At any given time, the ongoing social ties between humans affect physical health, including mental health – for better or worse.

The multidimensional construct of well being, understood not just as the absence of illness but as optimal psychosocial functioning across multiple domains, consistently emphasises the importance of social relationships for flourishing (Butler & Kern, 2016). The literature on affect, psychosocial well being, and health are voluminous, with robust connections between both negative and positive emotions and a range of health outcomes (Cohen & Pressman, 2006; DeSteno et al., 2013; Hernandez et al., 2018; Kubzansky et al., 2014; Suls, 2018).

Likewise, in recent years, a rapidly growing literature has developed on the importance of good quality social relationships or social ties for positive mental and physical health (Holt-Lunstad & Uchino, 2015; Umberson et al., 2010). Several articles provide consistent and compelling evidence that links the quality of social ties with a host of conditions, including the development and progression of cardiovascular disease, recurrent myocardial infarction, high blood pressure, cancer and delayed cancer recovery, and slower wound healing (Ertel et al., 2009; Everson-Rose & Lewis, 2005; Robles & Kiecolt-Glaser, 2003; Uchino, 2006). Still, other research studies have connected supportive interactions with others to benefit immune, endocrine, and cardiovascular functions (Seeman et al., 2002; Uchino, 2004).

Equally interesting are studies that show marital history shapes a range of health outcomes, including cardiovascular disease, chronic conditions, mobility limitations, and depressive symptoms (Hughes & Waite, 2009; Zhang & Hayward, 2006). Having children (Denney, 2010) is linked to positive health behaviours; however, marriage and parenthood have also been associated with behaviours (physical inactivity and weight gain) that are not beneficial to health. For example, marriage is the most salient source of both support and stress for many individuals (Walen & Lachman, 2000; Yang et al., 2014), and poor marital quality has been associated with compromised immune and endocrine function and depression (Kiecolt-Glaser & Newton, 2001). Sociological research shows that marital strain erodes physical health and that the negative effect of marital strain on health becomes more significant with advancing age (Umberson et al., 2006, 2010).

Caring for one's social relationships may also involve personal health costs. For example, providing care to a sick or impaired spouse imposes strains that undermine the provider's health (Christakis & Allison, 2006). Caring for a sick or impaired spouse is associated with increased physical and psychiatric morbidity, impaired immune function, and worse health for the provider (Schulz & Sherwood, 2008).

One of the largest and well-known studies is the Adverse Childhood Experiences (ACE) study, which describes the long-term relationship between childhood experiences and medical and public health problems (Felitti et al., 1998). This study identified stable family relationships as one of the key protective factors against adversity in childhood. A study by Brinker and Cheruvu (2017) found that social and emotional support can mitigate against the psychological distress associated with the experience of adverse childhood experiences and recommends interventions designed to promote social ties and relational connections that offer emotional support.

Protective factor of social support and STP

"Social support" refers to the emotionally sustaining qualities of relationships (e.g., a sense that one is loved, cared for, and listened to). With evidence showing that social relationships affect a range of health outcomes, interventions that decrease isolation and provide social support and education are beneficial as protective factors against challenging circumstances.

This brings us to how we envision STP as an intervention that connects group members socially with others and, as a result, provides opportunities for growth in biopsychosocial health and wellness. To understand how using STP can act upon these multilayered and interacting ecologies within social, psychological and biological processes, we return to our initial questions:

How do building models and sharing with others help make social connections?

Why do we see accelerated group cohesion during STP?

Why do these groups dive quite quickly into emotional expression?

How does building and sharing with others help make social connections?

Gargiulo (2005, p. 21) states, "the quickest path between yourself and another person is a story." By sharing our stories and listening to the stories of others, we are given the reciprocal opportunity to consider other perspectives. "Listening to stories encourages us to reflect on our similarities, appreciate other perspectives, and negotiate our differences" (p. 26).

When an STP group is formed around a health issue (coping with the pandemic, stress, mental health, physical disabilities, cancer, stroke-recovery), there is both the individual's sense-making process that occurs and a shared sense-making process that co-occurs. Being part of the group that has come together because of shared experiences, albeit unique and individualised, creates a sense of belonging.

Sharing of stories is the engine of STP, and quickly, participant stories create a sense of belonging and community sharing. Rimé (2018) studied the role of emotions, health, and well being regulated through the social sharing of emotional states. In his view, the necessarily private nature of our emotional states is stressful, and relief from that stress comes, in part, from making our internal emotional states known to our social community through the act of sharing. According to Rimé, sharing contributes to feelings of being known, reducing stress and promoting health. Rimé also noted that bonding and social cohesion increase when groups share.

In addition, it is highly likely that the STP participants are often at different points in their coping phases, which offers the opportunity for the mechanism of change factor of "the instillation of hope" to occur (Yalom & Leszcz, 2020). This instillation of hope allows group members to be inspired by others as they witness various ways in which others are coping with similar issues. Individuals can gain insight into how others gain awareness of ways to cope through the communally shared stories at different stages of a health journey.

Why do we see accelerated group cohesion during STP?

Group cohesiveness is another mechanism of change in the therapeutic application of LSP and is analogous to the relationship in individual therapy. Many relationships in a group are dynamically occurring, including intrapersonal, interpersonal, and group variables. The individual participant has a relationship with the group facilitator, other group members, and the group as a whole. All these relationships are what make up "group cohesiveness" and are interwoven with the story-sharing aspects of STP, and the playful nature of LEGO® building, the dimensions of flow, and the symbolism embedded in the STP process all combine as an accelerant to group cohesion.

Humans are social creatures, and they rely "on a safe, secure social surround to survive and thrive" (Hawkley & Cacioppo, 2010, p. 218). In STP, a group member may realise that they are not just passive beneficiaries of group cohesion but also generate that cohesion. Belonging and contributing to cohesion, even in a short-term group experience, can aid emotional connectedness, relationship building, and self-esteem (Yalom & Leszcz, 2020). Alternatively, skilled facilitators should be aware of "groupthink," where members might feel compelled to share the same beliefs or emotions of others when they actually do not. Facilitators should endorse respectful divergence of thought, risk-taking, and constructive expression of differences that, if done well, only enhance both emotional safety and group cohesiveness.

The STP facilitator must design the group experience as a lever for cohesion and interaction. Fortunately, the process of the traditional LSP model already has this built into its fabric. The learning experience creates space that maximises verbal collisions through visual storytelling and sharing. The powerful but simple rule that encourages, spotlights, and values full group contribution ensures everyone has a voice. The facilitator seeks out connections and makes sure voices are heard.

The potential impact of emotion sharing also occurs when individuals listen to others' stories (Curci & Bellelli, 2004; Harber & Cohen, 2005). Parkinson et al. (2005) concluded that, when participants experience similar emotions in response to emotional stories, their feeling of cohesion increases. Peters and Kashima (2007) observed that telling stories creates a partnership between the story narrator and the audience.

Why do these groups dive quite quickly into emotional expression?

As discussed in previous chapters, the use of metaphors and storytelling is fertile ground for emotional sharing. Researchers have discovered chemicals like cortisol, dopamine, and oxytocin are released in the brain when we tell or listen to stories (Brockington et al., 2021; Yuan et al., 2018). Cortisol assists with our formulating memories, and dopamine helps regulate our emotional responses that keep us engaged and in the moment. When it comes to creating deeper connections with others, oxytocin is associated with empathy – an essential element in building, deepening, or maintaining good relationships (Brockington et al., 2021).

The term "psychological safety" has been referred to in previous chapters and studied within the context of LSP (Grayburn, 2020; McCusker, 2020; Wheeler et al., 2020). The group facilitator is key to creating psychological safety and influences communication patterns by modelling behaviours such as timely self-disclosure and compassionate feedback. It is the facilitator's responsibility to treat the sharing of emotions in a group setting as hallowed ground.

When psychological safety is present, feeling expression is invited. Typical of many group-work-process experiences, emotional expression occurs when one participant takes the invitation and shares something personal or emotional through their brick model story. This seems to "give permission" to others to witness how the facilitator responds to the individual and group members. This interaction is called a vulnerability loop, coined by Dr Jeff Polzer, a professor of organisational behaviour at Harvard who studied how small, seemingly insignificant social exchanges in a group actually create tremendous impact (Coyle, 2018).

The loop refers to when an individual shares a moment of vulnerability. Then a second person detects the signal and recognises the first person's vulnerability by responding with their own vulnerability. Therefore, according to Coyle (2018), vulnerability is less about the sender of the initial message than the receiver. From this seemingly simple exchange, the shifting of the group dynamics occurs, and a norm is set that infers it is okay to admit weakness and help one another.

If the exchange is done well, the precedent is set, and the door is open to deeper sharing of emotionally laden content. Dependent on the participants' comfort level and the facilitator's skill, this initial occurrence broadens their willingness to share more emotionally laden descriptors in their metaphoric representations of their brick models and stories.

Given many health-related conditions, disorders, or experiences are often out of synchrony with the person's expectations, they are often tinged with emotion. This is often the case in STP, especially around health and well being topics. Emotion is stimulated as people share their experiences with others through their brick models. The psychosocial dynamic involved in both emotion sharing (Rimé, 2018) and self-disclosure (Reis & Patrick, 1996) ends up strengthening group social bonds

(Collins & Miller, 1994). In addition, repeatedly communicated emotional information enriches the social collective and provides them with shared knowledge, enabling them to cope more effectively with future emotional situations (Peters et al., 2009; Peters & Kashima, 2007).

Like many therapeutic encounters with a narrative component, the participants and the facilitator(s) become storykeepers (Goodyear-Brown, 2021). Not everyone has the skills intuitively to be a storykeeper, so the therapeutic skills of the STP facilitator are extremely critical to ensure the psychological safety of the group remains.

Conclusion

In this chapter, we extended the biopsychosocial model by adding Bronfenbrenner's (1979) human ecologies model and Berns' (2016) model of social systems to conceptualise how STP is positioned within these models. These integrative frameworks point to humans' interdependent social ecologies as contexts in which cognitive, affective, and physiological functions emerge and adapt. Given STP is an experience at the interpersonal, intrapersonal, and intragroup levels, in this chapter, we focussed on the role of social support in health. The interdependency of physical and mental health was highlighted to create a clear linkage or connection between physical and mental health. In doing so, we believe the constructs be considered together as one, not separate.

We examined the important role of social relationships in health – specifically, the protective factors that social support affords us during times of health concerns. Specific to STP, we focussed on the therapeutic applications of a group with a health focus, the key competencies of the facilitator, and why STP in groups has multiple benefits. We revisit answers to the questions of "how and why" STP impacts social connectedness, group cohesion, and accelerated emotional expression. Lastly, as STP continues to expand into various therapeutic applications, we believe our understanding of the interconnections will advance to greater and deeper levels.

References

Berns, R. M. (2016). *Child, family, school, community: Socialization and support* (10th ed.). Cengage Learning.

Brinker, J., & Cheruvu, V. K. (2017). Social and emotional support as a protective factor against current depression among individuals with adverse childhood experiences. *Preventive Medicine Reports, 5,* 127–133. https://doi.org/10.1016/j. pmedr.2016.11.018

Brockington, G., Gomes Moreira, A. P., Buso, M. S., Gomes da Silva, S., Altszyler, E., Fischer, R., & Moll, J. (2021). Storytelling increases oxytocin and positive emotions and decreases cortisol and pain in hospitalized children. *Proceedings of the National Academy of Sciences, 118*(22), e2018409118. https://doi.org/10.1073/ pnas.2018409118

Bronfenbrenner, U. (1979). *The ecology of human development: Experiments by nature and design.* Harvard University Press.

Bronfenbrenner, U. (1995). Developmental ecology through space and time: A future perspective. In P. Moen, G. H. Elder Jr., & K. Luscher (Eds.), *Examining lives in context: Perspectives on the ecology of human development* (pp. 619–647). American Psychological Association. https://doi.org/10.1037/10176-018

Bronfenbrenner, U. (2005). *Making human beings human: Bioecological perspectives on human development.* SAGE Publications.

Bronfenbrenner, U., & Morris, P. A. (2006). The bioecological model of human development. In I. W. Damon & R. M. Lerner (Eds.), *Handbook of child psychology* (Vol. 1, 6th ed.). John Wiley & Sons. https://doi.org/10.1002/9780470147658. chpsy0114

Butler, J., & Kern, M. L. (2016). The PERMA-Profiler: A brief multidimensional measure of flourishing. *International Journal of Wellbeing, 6*(3), 1–48. https://doi. org/10.5502/ijw.v6i3.526

Christakis, N., & Allison, P. (2006). Mortality after the hospitalization of a spouse. *The New England Journal of Medicine, 354*(7), 719–730. https://doi.org/10.1056/ NEJMsa050196

Cohen, S., & Pressman, S. D. (2006). Positive affect and health. *Current Directions in Psychological Science, 15,* 122–125. https://doi.org/10.1111/j.0963-7214.2006.00420.x

Collins, N. L., & Miller, L. C. (1994). Self-disclosure and liking: A meta-analytic review. *Psychological Bulletin, 116*(3), 457–475. https://doi.org/10.1037/ 0033-2909.116.3.457

Coyle, D. (2018). *The culture code.* Bantam Books.

Curci, A., & Bellelli, G. (2004). Cognitive and social consequences of exposure to emotional narratives: Two studies on secondary social sharing of emotions. *Cognition & Emotion, 18*(7), 881–900. https://doi.org/10.1080/02699930341000347

Denney, J. T. (2010). Family and household formations and suicide in the United States. *Journal of Marriage and Family, 72*(1), 202–213. https://doi. org/10.1111/j.1741-3737.2009.00692.x

DeSteno, D., Gross, J. J., & Kubzansky, L. (2013). Affective science and health: The importance of emotion and emotion regulation. *Health Psychology, 32,* 4744–4786. https://doi.org/10.1037/a0030259

Ertel, K. A., Glymour, M. M., & Berkman, L. F. (2009). Social networks and health: A life course perspective integrating observational and experimental evidence. *Journal of Social and Personal Relationships, 26*(1), 73–92. https://doi.org/10.1177/0265407509105523

Everson-Rose, S. A., & Lewis, T. T. (2005). Psychosocial factors and cardiovascular diseases. *Annual Review of Public Health, 26,* 469–500. https://doi.org/10.1146/annurev.publhealth.26.021304.144542

Felitti, V. J., Anda, R. F., Nordenberg, D., Williamson, D. F., Spitz, A. M., Edwards, V., Koss, M. P., & Marks, J. S. (1998). Relationship of childhood abuse and household dysfunction to many of the leading causes of death in adults: The adverse childhood experiences (ACE) study. *American Journal of Preventive Medicine, 14*(4), 245–258. https://doi.org/10.1016/s0749-3797(98)00017-8

Gargiulo, T. L. (2005). *The strategic use of stories in organizational communication and learning* (1st ed.). Routledge.

Goodyear-Brown, P. (2021). *Parents as partners in child therapy: A clinician's guide* (Illustrated ed.). The Guilford Press.

Grayburn, K. O. L. (2020). *Mindfulness and LEGO® SERIOUS PLAY®: How can the practice of mindfulness enhance the facilitation of LEGO® SERIOUS PLAY® workshops?* Independently Published.

Harber, K. D., & Cohen, D. J. (2005). The emotional broadcaster theory of social sharing. *Journal of Language and Social Psychology, 24*(4), 382–400. https://doi.org/10.1177/0261927X05281426

Hawkley, L. C., & Cacioppo, J. T. (2010). Loneliness matters: A theoretical and empirical review of consequences and mechanisms. *Annals of Behavioral Medicine, 40*(2), 218–227. https://doi.org/10.1007/s12160-010-9210-8

Hernandez, R., Bassett, S. M., Boughton, S. W., Schuette, S. A., Shiu, E. W., & Moskowitz, J. T. (2018). Psychological well-being and physical health: Associations, mechanisms, and future directions. *Emotion Review, 10*(1), 18–29. https://doi.org/10.1177/1754073917697824

Holt-Lunstad, J., & Uchino, B. N. (2015). Social support and health. In K. Glanz, B. K. Rimer, & K. V. Viswanath (Eds.), *Health behavior: Theory, research, and practice* (5th ed., pp. 183–204). Jossey-Bass/John Wiley & Sons.

Hughes, M. E., & Waite, L. J. (2009). Marital biography and health at mid-life. *Journal of Health and Social Behavior, 50*(3), 344–358. https://doi.org/10.1177/002214650905000307

Kiecolt-Glaser, J. K., & Newton, T. L. (2001). Marriage and health: His and hers. *Psychological Bulletin, 127*(4), 472–503. https://doi.org/10.1037/0033-2909.127.4.472

Kubzansky, L. D., Winning, A., & Kawachi, I. (2014). Affective states and health. In L. F. Berkman, I. Kawachi, & M. M. Glymour (Eds.), *Social epidemiology* (pp. 320–364). Oxford University Press. https://doi.org/10.1093/med/9780195377903.003.0009

McCusker, S. (2020). Everybody's monkey is important: LEGO® SERIOUS PLAY® as a methodology for enabling equality of voice within diverse groups. *International*

Journal of Research & Method in Education, 43(2), 146–162. https://doi.org/10.1 080/1743727X.2019.1621831

Moran, M. B., Frank, L. B., Zhao, N., Gonzalez, C., Thainiyom, P., Murphy, S. T., & Ball-Rokeach, S. J. (2016). An argument for ecological research and intervention in health communication. *Journal of Health Communication, 21*(2), 135–138. https://doi.org/10.1080/10810730.2015.1128021

Parkinson, B., Fischer, A., & Manstead, A. (2005). *Emotion in social relations: Cultural, group, and interpersonal processes.* Psychology Press. https://doi.org/10.4324/9780203644966

Peters, K., & Kashima, Y. (2007). From social talk to social action: Shaping the social triad with emotion sharing. *Journal of Personality and Social Psychology, 93*(5), 780–797. https://doi.org/10.1037/0022-3514.93.5.780

Peters, K., Kashima, Y., & Clark, A. (2009). Talking about others: Emotionality and the dissemination of social information. *European Journal of Social Psychology, 39*(2), 207–222. https://doi.org/10.1002/ejsp.523

Reis, H. T., & Patrick, B. C. (1996). Attachment and intimacy: Component processes. In *Social psychology: Handbook of basic principles* (pp. 523–563). The Guilford Press.

Rimé, B. (2018). Comment: Social integration and health: Contributions of the social sharing of emotion at the individual, the interpersonal, and the collective level. *Emotion Review, 10*(1), 67–70. https://doi.org/10.1177/1754073917719330

Robles, T. F., & Kiecolt-Glaser, J. K. (2003). The physiology of marriage: Pathways to health. *Physiology & Behavior, 79*(3), 409–416. https://doi.org/10.1016/S0031-9384(03)00160-4

Schulz, R., & Sherwood, P. R. (2008). Physical and mental health effects of family caregiving. *American Journal of Nursing, 108*(9), 23–27. https://doi.org/10.1097/01.NAJ.0000336406.45248.4c

Seeman, T. E., Singer, B. H., Ryff, C. D., Dienberg Love, G., & Levy-Storms, L. (2002). Social relationships, gender, and allostatic load across two age cohorts. *Psychosomatic Medicine, 64*(3), 395–406. https://doi.org/10.1097/00006842-200205000-00004

Suls, J. (2018). Toxic affect: Are anger, anxiety, and depression independent risk factors for cardiovascular disease? *Emotion Review, 10*(1), 6–17. https://doi.org/10.1177/1754073917692863

Uchino, B. N. (2004). *Social support and physical health: Understanding the health consequences of relationships.* Yale University Press. https://doi.org/10.12987/yale/9780300102185.001.0001

Uchino, B. N. (2006). Social support and health: A review of physiological processes potentially underlying links to disease outcomes. *Journal of Behavioral Medicine, 29*(4), 377–387. https://doi.org/10.1007/s10865-006-9056-5

Umberson, D., Crosnoe, R., & Reczek, C. (2010). Social relationships and health behavior across the life course. *Annual Review of Sociology, 36*(1), 139–157. https://doi.org/10.1146/annurev-soc-070308-120011

Umberson, D., Williams, K., Powers, D. A., Liu, H., & Needham, B. (2006). You make me sick: Marital quality and health over the life course. *Journal of Health and Social Behavior*, *47*(1), 1–16. https://doi.org/10.1177/002214650604700101

Walen, H. R., & Lachman, M. E. (2000). Social support and strain from partner, family, and friends: Costs and benefits for men and women in adulthood. *Journal of Social and Personal Relationships*, *17*(1), 5–30. https://doi.org/10.1177/0265407500171001

Wheeler, S., Passmore, J., & Gold, R. (2020). All to play for: LEGO® SERIOUS PLAY® and its impact on team cohesion, collaboration and psychological safety in organisational settings using a coaching approach. *Journal of Work-Applied Management*, *12*(2), 141–157. https://doi.org/10.1108/JWAM-03-2020-0011

Yalom, I. D., & Leszcz, M. (2020). *The theory and practice of group psychotherapy* (6th ed.). Basic Books.

Yang, Y. C., Schorpp, K., & Harris, K. M. (2014). Social support, social strain and inflammation: Evidence from a national longitudinal study of U.S. adults. *Social Science & Medicine*, *107*, 124–135. https://doi.org/10.1016/j.socscimed.2014.02.013

Yuan, Y., Major-Girardin, J., & Brown, S. (2018). Storytelling is intrinsically mentalistic: A functional magnetic resonance imaging study of narrative production across modalities. *Journal of Cognitive Neuroscience*, *30*(9), 1298–1314. https://doi.org/10.1162/jocn_a_01294

Zhang, Z., & Hayward, M. D. (2006). Gender, the marital life course, and cardiovascular disease in late midlife. *Journal of Marriage and Family*, *68*(3), 639–657. https://doi.org/10.1111/j.1741-3737.2006.00280.x

Chapter 8
When social and emotional systems play together
Mary Anne Peabody

As humans, we enter the world because of others, we survive because of others, and we benefit throughout our lives based on the actions of others. This interdependence on others extends across our life span. As social beings, the innate motivation for connection is deeply embedded in our biological makeup. We are born into a world with the help of others, we are dependent on others in our early years to survive, and, as research validates, those early childhood years create a strong foundation for social and emotional skill development that helps us develop and maintain healthy relationships and navigate stress through life (Bethell et al., 2017).

Humans, as social beings, are at the heart of every complex system, including our families, social groups, workplace relationships, community, and societal ecologies. At its most basic level, a system is a group of interrelated, interacting, or interdependent parts that form a unified whole working on a specific purpose. This is analogous to building with individual LEGO® bricks to create a 3-dimensional model in response to a purposeful question. The word "system" is derived from the Greek word *sunistánai*, meaning "to cause to stand together" (Williams, 2017, p. 18). The vital notion of togetherness in Williams' description implies that we should focus more on the dynamic relations between rather than the individual parts of any human system.

DOI: 10.4324/9781003260424-9

In this chapter, we suggest that having a "systems thinking" mindset as a Seriously Therapeutic Play with LEGO® (STP) facilitator can be beneficial to the success of the group and argue that the use of LEGO® within this mindset is a vital practice for skill development within the social and emotional learning (SEL) system. We will introduce the core competencies of social and emotional learning and then focus specifically on the skill of reflection that is embedded in the traditional LSP methodology but required within STP. We highlight the difference in STP, where the skill of reflection is targeted more often on self-reflection. This focus on self-reflection is a key distinguishing factor of the STP approach and includes feeling identification that leads to a deeper sense of self-awareness. We highlight pre-requisite or pre-conditional skills in self-reflection by presenting a "permissions model of reflective practice" that includes three broad domains: self-awareness, observation, effective communication, and six subskills (Peabody et al., 2022) as a guiding systems framework applicable for use in the in STP application.

Systems and connections

The influence of systems thinking on organisational strategic thinking and visioning is deeply embedded in the LEGO® SERIOUS PLAY® (LSP) process and its associated literature (Gauntlett, 2014; Kristiansen & Rasmussen, 2014; Oliver & Roos, 2000). Historically, the traditional LSP methodology was created from a worldview of organisational behaviour and operations within complex adaptive systems (Oliver & Roos, 2000). As the LSP facilitator guides participants through the seven applications of the full LSP methodology, participants see connections, patterns, and scenarios between organisational processes and the people working in the organisation (Kristiansen & Rasmussen, 2014). Furthermore, LSP participants are challenged to continuously think about the organisational structure, climate, situations, and events connected and at play throughout different systems. In fact, in later applications of the traditional LSP methodology, participants are led through a process of identification of specific systems and their impact (Kristiansen & Rasmussen, 2014). This includes envisioning emergent scenarios, strategies, and decisions about how the system is impacted by and responds to various events and choices (Kristiansen & Rasmussen, 2014).

Applying system thinking to the therapeutic application of LSP in the STP approach also has historical underpinnings; system approaches have been used for decades in approaches to treatment in family and group treatment (Bowen, 1978; Minuchin, 2012; Satir, 1967). Naturally, family and group systems organise themselves and create patterns of communication and behaviour (Connors & Caple, 2005). In the STP group, participants bring their own thinking and communication patterns based on their individual systems (families, community, society, workplace) as they interact with other group members and the facilitator. As STP participants form relationships, the group becomes an interactive system whereby patterns and interactional communication processes take place. In fact, the STP group itself functions as a system that takes on a life with its group members influencing the communication and behaviour of each other. Therefore, the group experience can be a fruitful training ground for social-emotional learning, social skill practice, and self-reflection.

Social and emotional learning as a system

The burgeoning field of social and emotional learning (SEL) has been gaining momentum for decades (Durlak et al., 2016). Depending on the context, various names may be used interchangeably to describe social and emotional learning, including emotional intelligence, emotional IQ, or interpersonal skills, to name a few. The terminology of social and emotional learning is often associated with children or youth, but the pandemic response to emotional and social needs across the lifespan highlighted that SEL is a human need across all developmental stages and in various contexts. For our purposes, we explore the current conceptual system of SEL and situate it within the STP experience.

Recently, the Collaborative for Social and Emotional Learning (CASEL, 2020) released the following definition, which has been adopted by many in the USA, Canada, and Australia. To ensure understanding of the terminology most commonly used, we share the following CASEL brief definitions. For more information, please explore the website at: www.panoramaed.com/blog/casel-new-definition-of-sel-what-you-need-to-know

Social and emotional learning (SEL) is integral to education and human development. SEL is the process through which all young people and adults acquire and apply the knowledge, skills, and attitudes to develop healthy identities, manage emotions and achieve personal and collective goals, feel and show empathy for others,

establish and maintain supportive relationships, and make responsible and caring decisions.

SEL advances educational equity and excellence through authentic school-family-community partnerships to establish learning environments and experiences that feature trusting and collaborative relationships, rigorous and meaningful curriculum and
instruction, and ongoing evaluation. SEL can help address various forms of inequity and empower young people and adults to
co-create thriving schools and contribute to safe, healthy, and just
communities.

From this definition, specific skills are further broken down into five categories: self-awareness, self-management, social awareness, relationship
skills, and responsible decision-making. The abilities and skills inherent
in the five areas touch upon both individual and social contexts and help
to create caring learning environments that are psychologically safe.

Beyond the definitions put forward by CASEL (2020), others (Goleman, 2014; Mayer et al., 2004) have identified interpersonal skill sets
similar to those mentioned earlier, including the abilities to detect voice
tones, read faces accurately, be empathic, actively listen well, and be
mindful of the emotions of others. Still, others (Kofman, 2014; Stone
et al., 1999) include the ability to communicate effectively, compromise,
engage in difficult conversations, and participate in respectful conflict
resolution.

Individuals who possess the interconnected social and emotional system of skills often find success with interpersonal relationships at work
and have positive mental health and overall increased well being (Bar-On
et al., 2006; Jordan & Ashkanasy, 2006; Lopes et al., 2005). All these
abilities are a life-long pursuit. Therefore, it behoves all of us to continuously practice these skills across the many systems we work, play, and live
in. We believe social-emotional learning and social skill development are
enhanced during STP when the facilitator directly creates time, space,
and attention to the pre-conditional skills of reflection.

Reflection and reflective practice

Reflection is a learned skill and a professional imperative across many
contexts. Reflection is a bridge linking knowledge of past, present, and

future; a skill or practice essential for life-long learning (Mckay, 2009). Scholars of reflective practice propose that, while an experiential activity is often considered the primary catalyst for learning, the actual learning occurs during reflective practice (Kolb & Kolb, 2005; Zigmont et al., 2011).

Dewey (1933), Schön (1983, 1987), Kolb (1984), and Brookfield (2017) have paved the way for the discussion of reflection and reflective practice. In both LSP and STP, the concepts put forth by Schon of "reflection in action" (looking at the present) and "reflection on action" (looking back) occur throughout the process. And with a future-oriented perspective, "reflection for action" is also considered (Cowan, 2020; Kinsella, 2001), as facilitators guide others to look forward while they imagine or anticipate the future based on current decisions and actions.

As reflection appears to be a common skill, it is easy to assume that people know how to intuitively reflect, which is often not the case. If STP facilitators hold this assumption, they may, unfortunately, fall into the trap of rushing through the "reflection" action phases (in-on-for) or not directly teach the skills. We believe reflection can be extended more broadly and deeply if facilitators clearly understand the pre-conditional skills and the importance of reflective questions that help participants find meaning. Facilitators have a responsibility to guide participants to reflect on their own and others' perspectives, stories, emotions, and decisions. These are the same core CASEL (2020) SEL skills definitions delineated earlier.

Reflection is the fourth core process step specific to LSP, where the facilitator guides participants to reflect on what they have heard and what they see in others' models but may not understand (Kristiansen & Rasmussen, 2014, p. 52). In STP, the focus is slightly different, with a focus on general reflection and an additional deeper, targeted, and more therapeutic focus on self-reflection. Self-reflection requires the individual to create a time and space for conscious introspection and reflection. Self-reflection is the extent to which an individual pays attention to and evaluates behaviours, feelings, and thoughts to clarify understanding (Grant et al., 2002).

We believe STP allows participants to have "permission to reflect," which opens up the ability for social learning to take place. We also believe there are pre-conditional skills that set the stage for effective self-reflection to take place, and several are naturally embedded into the

STP process. We now introduce a permissions model developed by one of the authors and colleagues (Peabody et al., 2022) using an adaptation of LSP that aligns nicely with our STP approach. The model is a conceptual frame to illustrate how pre-conditional, reflective practice skills can be taught indirectly and directly.

Permissions model: a focus on pre-requisite skills for group work using LSP

The permissions model includes three broad domains: self-awareness, observation, and effective communication and six pre-requisite skills, including permission for:

a)   Slowing down when necessary.
b)   Tolerating ambiguity.
c)   Noticing, thinking, and pondering.
d)   Speaking up.
e)   Listening with careful consideration of others' thinking.
f)   Respectfully building or challenging the ideas of others based on visual evidence.

The permissions model is influenced by Gibbs' (1988) reflective cycle model, which provides an integrative perspective that includes experiences, cognition, emotions, perception, and behavioural action. Gibbs' traditional reflective cycle encourages participants to think systematically about their experiences by posing key questions to guide their thinking. Individuals are asked to describe the event; ponder how they were feeling or what they were thinking about, then evaluate the event in terms of positives and challenges; make sense of the event and consider how they might act differently if the situation arose in the future. In STP, the focus is modified slightly; given the therapeutic nature of the objectives and goals, facilitators invite, encourage, prompt, and spend time in the space of "emotions and feelings" that are shared through the construction of the LEGO® models and the development of the narrative stories.

While the full explanation of the permissions model is beyond the scope of this chapter, for our purposes, a brief description of the components will be shared to illustrate the connections across systems of emotional-social learning, social skill development, and STP group experiences (Peabody et al., 2022; Figure 8.1).

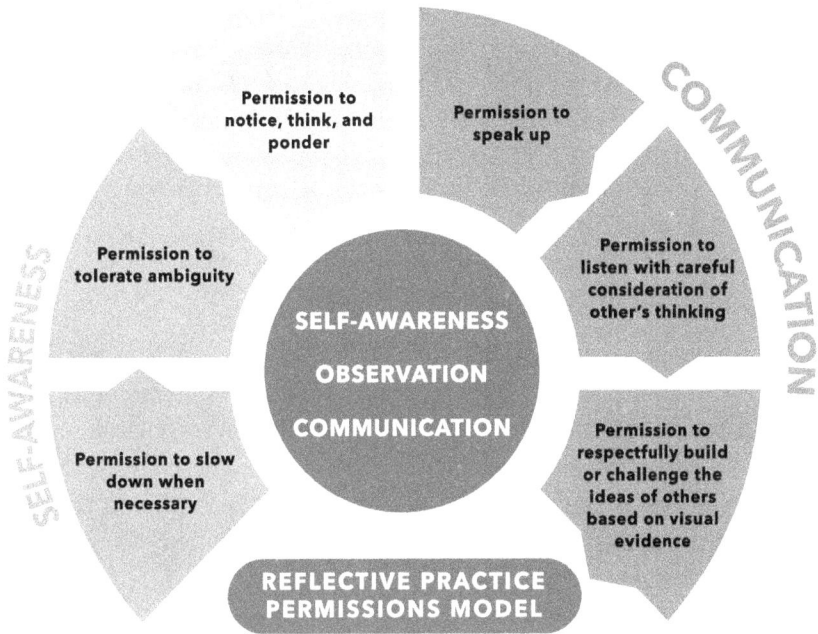

Figure 8.1 *Permissions model of reflective practice.*

The permissions model of reflective practice

It is important to note that, while the six permissions are broken down into separate components for visual ease, they do not occur in sequential order. The permission pre-skills often co-occur, making it an integrative model. For example, listening with careful consideration of others' thinking requires slowing down when necessary. Creating time and space for noticing, thinking, and pondering more deeply may build a tolerance for ambiguity and a sense of safety to speak up within the group. To respectfully challenge the thinking of others backed by visual evidence requires an openness to self-awareness and collegiality. When these permissions are carefully introduced, reinforced, and referred to throughout the group experience, the potential to impact and contribute to member reflective practice competency is greatly enhanced.

Self-awareness domain

Permission to slow down when necessary

One must slow down to engage in effective self-reflection. Slowing down, when necessary, allows participants time to consider their values, beliefs, and biases. Allowing this intentional slowing and time for reflection, participants may gain deeper insight into their experiences because simply having experiences will not necessarily bring new learning. Slowing down, when necessary, takes intentionality, as both individual and environmental barriers make slowing down difficult. The actual time taken in building the models also allows for some "slowing down" to think to be realised.

Permission to tolerate ambiguity

Not always having a clear direction or answer can be frustrating for many adults. By normalising ambiguity as part of complex systems, participants can reflect on their own discomfort and begin to self-regulate this emotional distress to allow for deeper reflection. These social skills are key for social competence in daily life. In many health-related therapeutic support groups, ambiguity around change and health are prevalent. Modelling the capacity for empathy around tolerating ambiguity can be important as a social skill to offer the group members.

Additionally, the permission to tolerate ambiguity is especially beneficial in the group-forming stage of the group. As mentioned in a previous chapter, the group provides a catalyst for social connectedness, group cohesion, and a sense of universality (Yalom & Leszcz, 2020). Participants can experience the reciprocal benefit of shared ambiguous experiences by helping and receiving help from others (Yalom & Leszcz, 2020).

Observation domain

Permission to notice, think, and ponder

This specific permission reminds participants that reflection is more than a cognitive process; it is an embodied process perceived through all our senses (Robinson, 2012). When group members notice how they feel, the impact of the feelings, and the role they play in a situation, they are once more engaging in self-awareness. Turning the step of noticing inward, individuals may discover their initial readings of a situation may have shifted shape, perspective, or intensity (James & Brookfield, 2014).

Building upon the "noticing" is the time to think and ponder what meaning exists from what is observed. This cognitive action allows meaning-making to occur and involves individuals connecting their past experiences with present occurrences by deliberately paying attention to themselves and others in the present moment. Several authors refer to this as being "mindful" and aware of what is happening within and around us (Grayburn, 2020; Hewson & Carroll, 2016; Siegel, 2007).

Communication domain

Permission to speak up

Equally important to observational skills is the ability to communicate observations accurately and effectively to others. Building further upon previous permissions, a participant must feel safe in the learning space to speak up, share thoughts, and be vulnerable. A supportive group climate involves creating an atmosphere that develops a sense of safety, freedom, and the comfort to share.

Speaking up to ask for help or clarification is a positive trait, and facilitators should work hard to instil this message and model it. Balancing time for all group members to share and ensuring no one dominates the communication process is built into the STP sequence of events through the process of moving from individual to shared builds.

Permission to listen with careful consideration of others' thinking

Permission to listen with careful consideration of others' thinking assumes that participants are skilled listeners; however, this may not be the case. Listening involves several fundamental components, such as attention to verbal and nonverbal communication, empathy, acceptance, and the ability to be nonjudgmental (Shipley, 2010).

Listening for understanding brings active listening to a deeper level and requires a range of subskills, including restating, reflecting, paraphrasing, pacing and silence, and feeling identification (Raskin et al., 2005). Depending on the group focus and goals, the listening skills for understanding may be explicitly focussed on with group participants or left more implicitly through modelling the skills through the facilitator's actions.

Permission to respectfully build upon or challenge the ideas of others based on visual evidence

This type of reflective practice encourages participants to show respect when building or expanding on someone's ideas or when challenging another participant. When offering an opposing perspective, participants are taught to provide evidence for their alternate perspective based on what they observe in the 3-D models to substantiate why they are making this claim. Ensuring alternative views or building upon the ideas of others must be facilitated and modelled clearly and respectfully to keep the overall psychological safety of the learning space at the forefront.

Reflection in, on, and for action

Revisiting the concepts put forward by Schön (1983, 1987) of "reflection in action" (looking at the present) and "reflection on action" (looking back) and Cowan (2020) and Kinsella (2001) of future-based action of "reflection for action," we consider when these different types of reflection occur. As participants share their brick models through stories and listen to others share, they enter the stage of "reflection in action." It is often during "reflection in action" that surprise arises as the usual assumptions or knowledge are challenged. As a facilitator, it is critical not to rush through this phase of reflection but rather to be patient and let the pace of the discovery unfold. The participants can gain many social and emotional learning opportunities by reflecting on themselves during the "reflection in action" phase. While "reflection in action" is embedded in the methodology, "reflection on action" that occurs in the final phase of the process deserves equal time and attention.

Once the participants stop building and sharing stories, the facilitator encourages them to think back about the overall building and sharing experience; in particular, to attend to their feelings and any meaning-making. As this phase is often last in the sequence of events, we have observed a number of concerns. This stage can easily be rushed through, superficially conducted, or dismissed altogether if a facilitator decides to move to the next application. This is less than ideal. Reflection on the entire STP experience deserves time and structure. We agree with Dewey when he stated, "We do not learn from experience, but from reflecting on experience." (1910/1933, p. 78).

Using or modifying a reflection model (Gibbs, 1988) that explores feelings or emotions is vitally important to the therapeutic aspects embedded in the STP approach and should be "at the forefront" in the facilitative process of the STP facilitator. Lastly, depending on the group, the facilitator can also weave "reflection for action" into the group discussion. "Reflection for action" focuses on future actions or behaviour and can be included as aspirational or future goal setting for participants. Reflection "in, on, and for" action builds participants' skills to become self-aware, keen observers, and effective communicators, all critical social and emotional skills for life.

Conclusion

The STP participants and facilitator form an interacting and interrelated micro-system where social and emotional learning is woven into the experience at each and every interaction. Facilitators play a critical role in creating a psychologically safe context for the preconditional skills to grow and permissions to engage in reflective practice are encouraged. Facilitators are also encouraged to avoid short-changing the importance of reflection on the overall process and to learn social competency skills in general.

Using a modification of Gibbs (1988) reflective cycle questions in a therapeutic application setting – along with the Permissions Model outlined (Peabody et al., 2022) – can provide a framework to augment growth in support of self-awareness, observation, and communication. As reflective facilitators, we can help others gain the vital skills that make being social beings a positive experience across and between the many systems in which we participate.

At the heart of the LEGO® System of play is an "everything connects to everything else" notion, beginning with the brick's interconnecting studs and tube system (Gauntlett, 2014). This connecting system can serve as a useful metaphor in explaining how the social experience of participating in the STP approach allows for ample opportunity to engage in self-reflection, leading to self- and other-awareness. These skills are all connected to having strong interpersonal relationships, both personally and professionally. We value having a "systems mindset" to help STP participants and facilitators see the interdependencies and connections across and between our relationships.

References

Bar-On, R., Handley, R., & Fund, S. (2006). *The impact of emotional intelligence on performance. In Linking emotional intelligence and performance at work: Current research evidence with individuals and groups* (pp. 3–19). Lawrence Erlbaum Associates Publishers.

Bethell, C. D., Carle, A., Hudziak, J., Gombojav, N., Powers, K., Wade, R., & Braveman, P. (2017). Methods to assess adverse childhood experiences of children and families: Toward approaches to promote child well-being in policy and practice. *Academic Pediatrics, 17*(7), S51–S69. https://doi.org/10.1016/j.acap.2017.04.161

Bowen, M. (1978). *Family therapy in clinical practice*. Rowman & Littlefield Publishers.

Brookfield, S. (2017). *Becoming a critically reflective teacher* (2nd ed.). John Wiley & Sons.

Collaborative for Social and Emotional Learning (CASEL). (2020). CASEL'S SEL frame-work. *CASEL*. https://casel.s3.us-east-2.amazonaws.com/CASEL-SEL-Framework-11.2020.pdf

Connors, J. V., & Caple, R. B. (2005). A review of group systems theory. *The Journal for Specialists in Group Work*, *30*(2), 93–110. https://doi.org/10.1080/01933920590925940

Cowan, J. (2020). Development of abilities begins from reflection-for-action. *Education & Self Development*, *15*(4), 9–20. https://doi.org/10.26907/esd15.4.04

Dewey, J. (1933). *How we think: A restatement of the relation of reflective thinking to the educative process*. D. C. Heath and Company. (Original work published 1910)

Durlak, J. A., Domitrovich, C., Weissberg, R. P., & Gullotta, T. P. (Eds.). (2016). *Handbook of social and emotional learning: Research and practice* (Paperback ed.). The Guilford Press.

Gauntlett, D. (2014). The LEGO system as a tool for thinking, creativity, and changing the world. In M. J. P. Wolf (Ed.), *LEGO studies: Examining the building blocks of a transmedial phenomenon* (pp. 189–205). Routledge. https://westminsterresearch.westminster.ac.uk/item/8yqq1/the-lego-system-as-a-tool-for-thinking-creativity-and-changing-the-world

Gibbs, G. (1988). *Learning by doing: A guide to teaching and learning methods*. Further Education Unit.

Goleman, D. (2014). *What makes a leader: Why emotional intelligence matters*. More Than Sound Publishing.

Grant, A. M., Franklin, J., & Langford, P. (2002). The self-reflection and insight scale: A new measure of private self-consciousness. *Social Behavior and Personality: An International Journal*, *30*(8), 821–835. https://doi.org/10.2224/sbp.2002.30.8.821

Grayburn, K. O. L. (2020). *Mindfulness and LEGO® SERIOUS PLAY®: How can the practice of mindfulness enhance the facilitation of LEGO® SERIOUS PLAY® workshops?* Independently Published.

Hewson, D., & Carroll, M. (2016). *Reflective practice in supervision*. Moshpit Publishing.

James, A., & Brookfield, S. D. (2014). *Engaging imagination: Helping students become creative and reflective thinkers* (1st ed.). Jossey-Bass.

Jordan, P. J., & Ashkanasy, N. M. (2006). Emotional intelligence, emotional self-awareness, and team effectiveness. In *Linking emotional intelligence and performance at work: Current research evidence with individuals and groups* (pp. 145–163). Lawrence Erlbaum Associates Publishers.

Kinsella, E. A. (2001). Reflections on reflective practice. *Canadian Journal of Occupational Therapy*, *68*(3), 195–198. https://doi.org/10.1177/000841740106800308

Kofman, F. (2014). *Authentic communication: Transforming difficult conversations in the workplace*. Sounds True.

Kolb, A. Y., & Kolb, D. A. (2005). Learning styles and learning spaces: Enhancing experiential learning in higher education. *Academy of Management Learning & Education*, *4*(2), 193–212. https://doi.org/10.5465/amle.2005.17268566

Kolb, D. A. (1984). *Experiential learning: Experience as the source of learning and development*. Prentice-Hall.

Kristiansen, P., & Rasmussen, R. (2014). *Building a better business using the LEGO® SERIOUS PLAY® method*. John Wiley & Sons.

Lopes, P. N., Salovey, P., Côté, S., & Beers, M. (2005). Emotion regulation abilities and the quality of social interaction. *Emotion*, *5*(1), 113–118. https://doi.org/10.1037/1528-3542.5.1.113

Mayer, J. D., Salovey, P., & Caruso, D. R. (2004). Emotional intelligence: Theory, findings, and implications. *Psychological Inquiry*, *15*(3), 197–215. https://doi.org/10.1207/s15327965pli1503_02

Mckay, E. (2009). Reflective practice: Doing, being and becoming a reflective practitioner. In E. A. S. Duncan (Ed.), *Skills for practice in occupational therapy* (pp. 55–72). Elsevier.

Minuchin, S. (2012). *Families and family therapy*. Harvard University Press.

Oliver, D., & Roos, J. (2000). *Striking a balance: Complexity and knowledge landscapes*. McGraw-Hill.

Peabody, M. A., Noyes, S., & Anderson, M. (2022). Permission to learn: Intentional use of art and object-mediated strategies to develop reflective professional skills. *Journal of Occupational Therapy Education*, *6*(3). https://doi.org/10.26681/jote.2022.060314

Raskin, N. J., Rogers, C. R., Corsini, R. J., & Wedding, D. (2005). Person-centered therapy. In *Current psychotherapies* (7th ed., pp. 130–165). Thomson Brooks/Cole Publishing Co. https://doi.org/10.1177/009318530403200411

Robinson, S. K. (Ed.). (2012). *Out of our minds: Learning to be creative*. John Wiley & Sons. https://doi.org/10.1002/9780857086549

Satir, V. (1967). *Conjoint family therapy: A guide to theory and technique* (Rev. ed.). Science and Behavior Books.

Schön, D. A. (1983). *The reflective practitioner: How professionals think in action*. Basic Books.

Schön, D. A. (1987). *Educating the reflective practitioner*. Jossey-Bass.

Shipley, S. D. (2010). Listening: A concept analysis. *Nursing Forum*, *45*(2), 125–134. https://doi.org/10.1111/j.1744-6198.2010.00174.x

Siegel, D. J. (2007). *The mindful brain: Reflection and attunement in the cultivation of well-being*. W. W. Norton & Company.

Stone, D., Patton, B., Heen, S., & Fisher, R. (1999). *Difficult conversations: How to discuss what matters most*. Penguin Books.

Williams, S. J. (2017). *Improving healthcare operations: The application of lean, agile and legality in care pathway design* (1st ed., 2017 ed.). Palgrave Pivot.

Yalom, I. D., & Leszcz, M. (2020). *The theory and practice of group psychotherapy* (6th ed.). Basic Books.

Zigmont, J. J., Kappus, L. J., & Sudikoff, S. N. (2011). The 3d model of debriefing: Defusing, discovering, and deepening. *Seminars in Perinatology, 35*(2), 52–58. https://doi.org/10.1053/j.semperi.2011.01.003

CHAPTER 9
CLUTCH POWER
WHEN THERAPEUTIC POWERS CONNECT

Mary Anne Peabody

The snapping noise that you hear when two LEGO® bricks are joined together is referred to as "clutch power," illustrating the remarkable strength of the interlocking connection between the tubes on the bottom of the bricks with the studs on top of the other bricks (Anthony, 2018; Skahill, 2020). This clutch power connection is part of the appealing genius in the overall design of the LEGO® system of play. In this chapter, we borrow the "clutch power" metaphor to describe the connective strength that emerges from the convergence of the therapeutic factors inherent in group work (Yalom & Leszcz, 2020) with the therapeutic factors of play (Schaefer & Drewes, 2014).

Therapeutic change is a complex process, and to approach this complexity, we examine the basic components of several therapeutic factors that are most prominent in the Serious Therapeutic Play with LEGO® (STP) approach. As we learnt in previous chapters, several integrated theoretical approaches underpin STP; therefore, if we combine the strength of both play and group factors, each potentiates the other's effects. Just as one brick connects to another through the element of clutch power, so, too, does STP have the power to hasten connections, enhance social learning, and accelerate emotional content making the group experience an impactful process for change and growth.

DOI: 10.4324/9781003260424-10

Therapeutic factors are defined as the mechanisms of change that occur through an intrinsic interplay of various guided human experiences (Yalom & Leszcz, 2020, p. 3). This definition is of great relevance to us, as it includes the word "interplay," denoting an active, reciprocal effect. If the components of the therapeutic exchange were placed on a continuum, therapeutic factors would lie in the middle, situated between theories and techniques (Schaefer & Drewes, 2014). Understanding these change factors in the context of group therapeutic work gives the therapist a rational basis for selecting strategies or tactics that shape the group experience (Yalom & Leszcz, 2020).

Yalom was one of the first to systematically study the factors triggering and enhancing the therapeutic change process in group psychotherapy, resulting in his model of 11 therapeutic factors (Barlow et al., 2000; Kivlighan & Arseneau, 2009; Yalom & Leszcz, 2020). The list was further expanded upon by others (Baourda, 2013; Bloch et al., 1979). However, this chapter will refer to the 11 factors Yalom and Leszcz (2020) used in the literature.

Likewise, Schaefer (1993) was the first to present 14 therapeutic factors of play, later expanding to 20 factors. These therapeutic factors are also referred to as "therapeutic powers of play" and were conceptualised based on accumulating literature, nascent research, and clinical experiences (Drewes & Schaefer, 2014). More recently, the United States Association of Play Therapy (2021) recognised the therapeutic factors/powers of play as foundational competency knowledge in the credentialing process of becoming a registered play therapist (Turner et al., 2020). While alternate definitions and characterisations of the therapeutic factors of play exist (O'Connor & Vega, 2019; Russ, 2004; Shirk & Russell, 1996), for purposes of this chapter, the categories from Drewes and Schaefer's model are utilised. A detailed exploration of all factors across both play and therapeutic group work is beyond the scope of this chapter. Readers are encouraged to become well versed in the literature surrounding the therapeutic factors that guide clinical decision-making.

As the biopsychosocial framework guides our book, it is critical to recognise the transtheoretical nature of STP and the need for an integrative approach. The trend towards integration is not new and is recognised by clinicians across various approaches, including those with a play-based affiliation (Drewes, 2009; Gil, 2015; Goodyear-Brown, 2010; Stricker & Gold, 2003). Therefore, it is incumbent for practitioners to understand the contributions of – and be trained in – several transtheoretical therapeutic models so they can effectively select, tailor, and integrate the models and factors to the group's unique needs.

In this chapter, we first describe the therapeutic factors of therapeutic group work and play, followed by a deeper exploration of the need for integration in therapeutic models. Next, we select and explore several therapeutic factors that are activated through STP. We recognise that other therapeutic factors could be further examined. The ones chosen will likely overlap, depending on the group being conducted and the participants involved, as interdependence is often occurring. Finally, we conclude with suggestions for practitioners to consider utilising therapeutic factors within the STP application process in their clinical reasoning.

The therapeutic factors of group work

Therapeutic factors are considered to emerge in all types of groups and therapeutic contexts, signifying a positive effect on the members' progress (Yalom & Leszcz, 2020). Originally, Yalom (1970) presented several therapeutic group work factors as mechanisms of change, and more recently, Yalom and Leszcz (2020) have identified the following 11 primary factors. A brief description of the terminology is offered.

- Instillation of hope: a sense of optimism about one's potential progress. Because group members are in different places along their paths of health or healing, they often naturally inspire each other and thereby help others with a sense of hopefulness.
- Universality: a recognition that one's experiences, feelings, and concerns are shared with others. Universality tends to normalize and validate experiences and helps participants connect and not feel so alone.
- Imparting information: all group members bring knowledge to the group. Through the process of sharing over time, group members gain valuable information about available resources and other useful facts both from one another and from the therapist.
- Altruism: the experience that group members are willing to help, support, and reassure others as group members. Participants benefit in a reciprocal, or give-and-take, manner, helping others and receiving help from others.
- Corrective recapitulation of the primary family group: group members often bond in ways reminiscent of relationships they

shared within their families. This experience may bring a range of emotions. The therapist must balance what is occurring in the here-and-now and what occurred in the past in other contexts for supportive and corrective therapeutic experiences that might lead to insight, healing, and growth.

- Development of socializing techniques: inherent in the social nature of groups, group members can develop a range of social skills, such as listening and responding, trusting others, impulse control, coping skills, appropriate conflict resolution, and experimenting with alternative expressions of emotions and behaviour.
- Imitative behaviour: group members learn by observation and then may attempt to copy the behaviour of the therapist and other group members.
- Interpersonal learning: in groups, the interpersonal efforts to relate constructively and adaptively are plentiful. Learning can occur through the observation of others or by discovering something significant about oneself. Interpersonal learning occurs in numerous ways, including the connections made individually and as a group, receiving feedback, advice, or suggestions from group members and therapists.
- Group cohesiveness: groups go through their own growth process over time, culminating in a sense that we are "in this together." Group work often bestows a sense of belonging, which meets a fundamental human need: the group "clicks."
- Catharsis: the group experience can serve as an emotional container for positive and negative emotions. When group members share their feelings and stories, they may feel a sense of release and, therefore, emotionally lighter.
- Existential factors: group work often promotes the experience that we are responsible for our actions and the consequences of our actions.

The therapeutic powers of play

Parsons (2021) compares the therapeutic powers of play to the catalyst properties of bodily enzymes that aid in the digestion of emotional material while facilitating movement towards optimal psychosocial and emotional health and overall well being. Drewes and Schaefer's (2014) categorical model is presented later under four broad domains: facilitates communication, fosters emotional wellness, increases personal strengths, and enhances social competence. Additionally, the model was intended to be re-examined over time as more process research on the therapeutic factors of play was conducted.

Facilitates communication

- Self-expression: play objects or play behaviour help communicate, verbally or non-verbally, ideas, thoughts, experiences, and emotions. The use of play-based metaphors helps express difficult feelings or narratives with the support and guidance of the therapist.
- Access to the unconsciousness: play-based fantasy, imagination, and metaphors often represent outside-of-awareness experiences. Play offers a way to tap into the unconscious and bring emotions and thoughts into conscious awareness.
- Direct teaching: play can explicitly teach content and specific skills. Games, role-play, bibliotherapy, and psychoeducation are examples of how play materials can explicitly teach information.
- Indirect teaching: play also allows knowledge and skills deficits to be addressed through implicit means. Imaginative play, fantasy, or pretend play, and storytelling with metaphors enable narratives to be told through representational and symbolic means.

Fosters emotional wellness

- Catharsis: a release of pent-up, negative emotions that offers stress-reducing potential. Play objects and play actions can allow negative experiences or feelings to be acted out and assist in pairing or labelling the action with the appropriate emotions.
- Abreaction: a heightened affective process often used with trauma reactions. A mechanism whereby mentally undigested traumatic experiences can be re-enacted and assimilated through the protective distance that metaphors, objects, or toys afford. This process can lead to a sense of control, increased insight, and a sense of mastery.
- Positive emotions: play offers a space to have fun and to engage in experiences that elicit laughter, smiles, happiness, and joy. These experiences are considered antidotes to more uncomfortable affects such as anxiety and depression (Schaefer, 1999).

- Counterconditioning fears: this power refers to the reducing or extinguishing of anxious or fearful responses by helping learn an incompatible response. Pairing the feared response with a playful counter-response can potentially weaken the feared response while simultaneously allowing for mastery or control.
- Stress inoculation: a preventative or rehearsal approach that uses play in advance of a stressful event. The anticipatory anxiety of a time-limited upcoming, stressful life event, such as a family move, starting school, or a medical visit, can be lessened by playing out the event before the actual event. Playing with miniature toys or objects can make the unfamiliar familiar and less scary, and strategies for coping can be modelled.
- Stress management: neuroscience has connected play with a reduction in our body's stress response (Bernard & Dozier, 2010). Using playful opportunities that often elicit laughter or engage in humorous moments allows a variety of physical and psychological benefits to occur, thereby releasing endorphins and decreasing blood pressure (Abel, 2002; Schaefer & Drewes, 2011).

Increases personal strengths

- Creative problem solving: play is rich in opportunities for exploration, creativity, and discovery. Fantasy or imaginative play requires creativity and divergent thinking. The ability to generate and explore novel and alternate solutions is associated with divergent thinking in fantasy play (Russ & Schafer, 2006).
- Resiliency: the ability or capacity to withstand, adapt, or rebound from challenging or disruptive life circumstances. Play experiences offer multiple opportunities to create a stronger sense of self.
- Moral development: specific types of play, such as game play or group play, are rich in opportunities to discuss right and wrong, winning and losing, and promote moral decision making associated with societal citizenship.
- Accelerated development: play develops a holistic array of skills across cognitive, linguistic, social, and emotional domains (Drewes & Schaefer, 2014; Moyles, 2005). The more play opportunities a child is offered, the greater the likelihood of holistic benefits (Hoffmann & Russ, 2012).
- Self-regulation: self-regulation is the skill of managing our thinking, feeling, and behaviour. The skills include cognitive flexibility,

self-monitoring, response inhabitation, and self-talk, and they can guide and help regulate our actions and synchronise our social behaviour with others (Barkley, 1997).

- Self-esteem: the sum of all a person can call their own across cognitive, affective, and behavioural domains: the physical self, psychological traits, feelings, family, friends, significant others, possessions, vocation, spiritual, hobbies. A sense of self can be developed through play experiences.

Enhances social relationships

- Therapeutic relationship: a fundamental transtheoretical element across many forms of psychotherapy that allows for psychological safety in the formation of interactions to accomplish therapeutic goals. The positive effects trigged in play connect us to one another and serve as the foundation for forming relational connections in psychotherapy.
- Attachment: play is how early relationships are formed in parent-child interactions and allows for active engagement leading to therapeutic progress. Play is how therapists can become emotionally close to clients.
- Social competence: a combination of desirable social skills that include communication, self-control of emotions and behaviour, and reciprocity with others. Socio-dramatic, rough-and-tumble play, and game play all embed social skill elements.
- Empathy: a complex neurobiological process that involves attention, reasoning to notice, observation, memory, knowledge, and the ability to comprehend and respond sensitively to the thoughts and feelings of others (Decety & Lamm, 2006). Empathy is a core skill in therapy and significantly influences therapeutic outcomes (Decety, 2011).

A need for integration

As discussed in previous chapters, STP has its roots in several different theories. Many helping professions recognise the need for and importance of adopting an integrative stance in assisting in managing human beings' complex needs (Kaduson et al., 2020). The psychological needs of those seeking therapeutic support are multi-layered and multi-determined, requiring an integrative approach. Integration is not random; it is the purposeful and flexible weaving of theory, therapeutic factors, and techniques across therapies.

Psychotherapy integration has a long and rich history (Seymour, 2011) and is commonly practised in adult and child therapeutic settings (Drewes, 2011; Norcross & Goldfried, 2005). Prochaska and Norcross (2010, p. 455) describe the motivation of psychotherapy integration as "a spirit of open inquiry and a zest for transtheoretical dialogue." An integrative approach espouses that psychological challenges have multiple biopsychosocial causes. There is rarely a "right" therapeutic method or one list of therapeutic factors appropriate in all situations; there are "many ways to health" (Lambert et al., 2004, p. 809). "An integrated multi-component intervention reflects the fact that most psychological disorders are complex and multidimensional, that is, they are caused by an interaction of biological, psychological and social factors" (Schaefer, 2011, p. 367).

Given that our book is conceptualised from a biopsychosocial perspective, we firmly believe the STP model represents a systematic integration of theoretical constructs, therapeutic factors of change, and techniques drawn from diverse schools of thought. Integrating LEGO® therapeutic play into the therapeutic realm adds to our therapeutic practice's "clutch power." We believe the clutch power of STP adds a powerful and robust approach to our therapeutic work. STP assists us to further integrate our understanding of psychology, behavioural sciences, education, and neuroscience, along with the mechanisms of therapeutic change, which produce the accelerating and amplification effect of successful therapy for change and growth (Peabody & Noyes, 2017).

Specific to the therapeutic factors of change, the literature reveals the existence of common factors across several approaches (Norcross & Goldfried, 2005; Wampold & Imel, 2015). Looking at the identified factors in the play and group work listings, one immediately sees similarities, albeit slightly varying terms. For example, social competence is analogous to the development of socialising techniques and interpersonal learning. Direct teaching is akin to imparting information. However, there are also spaces of distinction, as therapeutic change can occur without play and therapeutic change mechanisms of play can occur without the context of a group experience.

In addition, utilising STP adds a kinaesthetic component paired with the metaphoric storymaking approach to elicit meaning-making. As previously discovered in earlier chapters, this tactile experience with our hands and the bricks activates different neurobiological processes adding a multidimensional aspect. Within the STP model, both common and specific therapeutic factors are valuable. However, it behoves the therapist to understand and utilise specific factors and tailor the therapeutic experience to the clients' unique needs, the type of group, and the therapeutic goals.

Conceptualising STP through the lens of therapeutic factors

Next, we apply the "therapeutic factors" conceptual lens to the STP approach. The task of the STP therapist is to ensure the appropriate integration of both play and change processes to meet the therapeutic goals. For clarity, I have highlighted the factors in italics.

STP operates within the context of a dynamic *relationship* that forms between the therapist and client(s) and between the group members themselves. LEGO® bricks are a core object of focus and tool for developing personal and group metaphors. The use of "bricks" elicits a playful side to the experiences that typically translate into a *positive emotional* experience. The communicative power of play is the cornerstone of the approach, so storytelling and storymaking in STP are rooted in *self-expression*.

The encouragement of symbolism and metaphor is unique to the building and storytelling/storymaking process. The use of bricks and metaphor deepens and decreases self-focus, providing the builder with a bit of distance and the power and choice to share or not to share. Given each group member selects and builds from a pile of bricks, their model and the accompanying story has unique meaning for the builder. The participant owns the story, its meaning, and how much they desire to share. This control and empowerment speak to an individual's *self-esteem* boosting potential that occurs when being seen and heard by others. In addition, if one feels validated or discovers that others may feel similarly, a sense of *universality* may develop, where, despite the uniqueness of individual stories, the phenomenon of being connected, "all in the same boat," can be healing and supportive. A skilled therapist titrates this sharing through their comments, responses, and pacing, thereby keeping a safe environment for all.

As participants build and share, their inner world is made visible. Sometimes the builds and the metaphors tap into *unconscious awareness* and help bring the internal out to the external world. Metaphors become the bridge to something difficult to say or memories or information not fully integrated into the individual's awareness (Dunn-Fierstein, 2013, p. 135). Through listening to the stories of others, participants develop the ability to see things from another's perspective, a core component of *empathy*. Sharing the space with others as they share emotional content deepens the ability to be "present" with others. It validates their narrative, and the therapist models the dance between empathic curiosity and invasiveness by focusing on the bricks and the associated metaphors rather than the individual, staying ever present with the therapeutic process.

Depending on the nature of the group (psychoeducation or support), there will be an *imparting of information* and, typically, a mix of *direct and indirect teaching*. For example, simply waiting during the story sharing of the STP process can teach *social competence* and develop *socialising techniques* such as impulse control, patience, and active listening skills. Direct teaching of stress reduction, pacing techniques, and reflection skills specific to the therapeutic challenges or diagnosis can be utilised in the prompts used in building and discussing the brick models. Simply listening and observing how the therapist paces the group experiences, responds with validation and encouragement, and asks open-ended questions allows group members to imitate and model appropriate behaviour. Over time, this often turns into experiences of *altruism*, where the reciprocal validation of feelings and experiences occurs.

Humans seem to grow and change when they give to others. Providing support and encouragement to others helps with isolation and creates a sense of group connection, belonging or *cohesion*. The experience of both giving and receiving validation is impactful and strengthens the group experience. Similarly, hearing similar stories can create a sense of *universality*, unique in group work where, although each member is different and unique in their stories, they can experience the phenomenon of connection, "all in the same boat," which can be healing.

Conclusion

In the world of LEGO®, every individual brick can connect to another. The clutch power first described by Godtfred Kirk Christiansen (Anthony, 2018; Skahill, 2020) changed the course of LEGO® as a toy and as a company and speaks to the remarkable strength of the interconnectedness between bricks to create a surprisingly solid structure.

This interconnectedness or interplay is also active in STP. This chapter integrated the therapeutic factors, the mechanisms of change, inherent in group work and play that most align with the therapeutic application of STP. Depending on the group makeup, goals, and intent, some therapeutic factors will connect, and others will not. What remains critical is that the facilitator has the knowledge and skill to use theory, facilitate therapeutic change, and apply the specific techniques that create the unique clutch power strength-based connections built via STP.

References

Abel, M. H. (2002). Humor, stress, and coping strategies. *International Journal of Humor Research*, *15*(4). https://doi.org/10.1515/humr.15.4.365

Anthony, W. (2018). The LEGO story. *Scandinavian Review*, 17–33.

Association for Play Therapy. (2021). *Credentialing standards for the registered play therapist: APT professional credentialing program*. www.a4pt.org/page/CredentialsHomepage

Baourda, V. C. (2013). *Group processes during a psychoeducational program for elementary school students with social anxiety* [Master's thesis, University of Ioannina].

Barkley, R. A. (1997). Behavioral inhibition, sustained attention, and executive functions: Constructing a unifying theory of ADHD. *Psychological Bulletin*, *121*(1), 65–94. https://doi.org/10.1037/0033-2909.121.1.65

Barlow, S. H., Burlingame, G. M., & Fuhriman, A. (2000). Therapeutic applications of groups: From Pratt's "thought control classes" to modern group psychotherapy. *Group Dynamics: Theory, Research, and Practice*, *4*(1), 115–134. https://doi.org/10.1037/1089-2699.4.1.115

Bernard, K., & Dozier, M. (2010). Examining infants' cortisol responses to laboratory tasks among children varying in attachment disorganization: Stress reactivity or return to baseline? *Developmental Psychology*, *46*(6), 1771–1778. https://doi.org/10.1037/a0020660

Bloch, S., Reibstein, J., Crouch, E., Holroyd, P., & Themen, J. (1979). A method for the study of therapeutic factors in group psychotherapy. *British Journal of Psychiatry*, *134*(3), 257–263. https://doi.org/10.1192/bjp.134.3.257

Decety, J. (2011). Dissecting the neural mechanism mediating empathy. *Emotion Review*, *3*(1), 92–108. https://doi.org/10.1177/1754073910374662.

Decety, J., & Lamm, C. (2006). Human empathy through the lens of social neuroscience. *The Scientific World Journal*, *6*, 1146–1163. https://doi.org/10.1100/tsw.2006.221

Drewes, A. A. (2009). Rationale for integrating play therapy and CBT. In A. A. Drewes (Ed.), *Blending play therapy with cognitive behavioral therapy: Evidence-based and other effective treatments and techniques* (pp. 1–2). John Wiley & Sons.

Drewes, A. A. (2011). Integrating play therapy theories into practice. In A. A. Drewes, S. C. Bratton, & C. E. Schaefer (Eds.), *Integrative play therapy* (pp. 21–35). John Wiley & Sons. https://doi.org/10.1002/9781118094792

Drewes, A. A., & Schaefer, C. E. (2014). Introduction: How play therapy causes therapeutic change. In *The therapeutic powers of play: 20 core agents of change* (2nd ed., pp. 1–8). John Wiley & Sons.

Dunn-Fierstein, P. (2013). Metaphorical language in sandplay therapy. *Journal of Sandplay Therapy*, *22*(1), 133–143.

Gil, E. (2015). *Play in family therapy* (2nd ed.). Guilford Press.

Goodyear-Brown, P. (2010). *Play therapy with traumatized children: A prescriptive approach*. John Wiley & Sons.

Hoffmann, J., & Russ, S. (2012). Pretend play, creativity, and emotion regulation in children. *Psychology of Aesthetics, Creativity, and the Arts*, *6*(2), 175–184. https://doi.org/10.1037/a0026299

Kaduson, H. G., Schaefer, C. E., & Cangelosi, D. (2020). Basic principles and core practices of prescriptive play therapy. In H. E. Kaduson, D. Cangelosi, & C. E. Schaefer (Eds.), *Prescriptive play therapy* (pp. 3–13). Guilford Press.

Kivlighan, D. M., & Arseneau, J. R. (2009). A typology of critical incidents in intergroup dialogue groups. *Group Dynamics: Theory, Research, and Practice*, *13*(2), 89–102. https://doi.org/10.1037/a0014757

Lambert, M. J., Bergin, A. E., & Garfield, S. L. (2004). Overview, trends and future issues. In M. J. Lambert (Ed.), *Bergin and Garfield's handbook of psychotherapy and behaviour change* (5th ed., pp. 805–821). John Wiley & Sons.

Moyles, J. (2005). *The excellence of play*. Open University Press.

Norcross, J. C., & Goldfried, M. R. (2005). *Handbook of psychotherapy integration* (2nd ed.). Oxford University Press.

O'Connor, K., & Vega, C. (2019). Ecosystemic play therapy. *Play Therapy*, *14*(3), 32–34.

Parson, J. (2021). Children speak play: Landscaping the therapeutic powers of play. In E. Prendiville & J. A. Parson (Eds.), *Clinical applications of therapeutic powers of play*. Routledge.

Peabody, M. A., & Noyes, S. (2017). Reflective boot camp: Adapting LEGO® SERIOUS PLAY® in higher education. *Reflective Practice*, *18*(2), 232–243. https://doi.org/10.1080/14623943.2016.1268117

Prochaska, J. O., & Norcross, J. C. (2010). *Systems of psychotherapy: A transtheoretical analysis* (7th ed.). Cole.

Russ, S. W. (2004). *Play in child development and psychotherapy: Toward empirically supported practice* (pp. xi, 181). Lawrence Erlbaum Associates Publishers.

Russ, S. W., & Schafer, E. D. (2006). Affect in fantasy play, emotion in memories, and divergent thinking. *Creativity Research Journal*, *18*(3), 347–354. https://doi.org/10.1207/s15326934crj1803_9

Schaefer, C. E. (1993). *The therapeutic powers of play*. Aronson.

Schaefer, C. E. (1999). Curative factors in play therapy. *The Journal for the Professional Counselor*, *14*, 7–16.

Schaefer, C. E. (2011). Prescriptive play therapy. In C. E. Schaefer (Ed.), *Foundations of play therapy* (pp. 2, 365–378). Wiley.

Schaefer, C. E., & Drewes, A. A. (2011). The therapeutic powers of play and play therapy. In *Foundations of play therapy* (2nd ed., pp. 15–25). John Wiley & Sons.

Schaefer, C. E., & Drewes, A. A. (Eds.). (2014). *The therapeutic powers of play: 20 core agents of change* (2nd ed.). John Wiley & Sons.

Seymour, J. W. (2011). History of psychotherapy integration and related research. In A. A. Drewes, S. C. Bratton, & C. E. Schaefer (Eds.), *Integrative play therapy* (pp. 3–19). John Wiley & Sons.

Shirk, S., & Russell, R. (1996). *Change processes in child psychotherapy: Revitalizing treatment and research*. Guilford Press.

Skahill, S. (2020). Surprising discovery about Godtfred Kirk Christiansen revealed on his 100th birthday. *LEGO Ambassador Network*. https://lan.lego.com/news/overview/surprising-discovery-about-godtfred-kirk-christiansen-revealed-on-his-100th-birthday-r265/

Stricker, G., & Gold, J. (2003). Integrative approaches to psychotherapy. In A. S. Gurman & S. B. Messer (Eds.), *Essential psychotherapies* (pp. 317–349). Guilford Press.

Turner, R., Schoeneberg, C., Ray, D., & Lin, Y.-W. (2020). Establishing play therapy competencies: A Delphi study. *International Journal of Play Therapy*, *29*(4), 177–190. https://doi.org/10.1037/pla0000138

Wampold, B. E., & Imel, Z. E. (2015). *The great psychotherapy debate: The evidence for what makes psychotherapy work*. (2nd ed.). Routledge; cat00097a. https://doi.org/10.4324/9780203582015

Yalom, I. D. (1970). *The theory and practice of group psychotherapy*. Basic Books.

Yalom, I. D., & Leszcz, M. (2020). *The theory and practice of group psychotherapy* (6th ed.). Basic Books.

CHAPTER 10

BUILDING SOCIALLY AND EMOTIONALLY
FROM ME TO WE

Mary Anne Peabody

Emotions play a critical role in our daily lives, influencing how we establish, maintain, and regulate social relationships. Relevant literature around the role of emotions in change efforts has been studied across multiple disciplines, and an overwhelming majority of authors now contend that individual and organisational change is fundamentally about emotions (Issah, 2018; Seijts & O'Farrell, 2003; Watkins et al., 2017). Emotions are not viewed as a cause of interference with the change process; rather, emotions are essential to it (Turesky & Peabody, 2018). In our STP approach, we assert that emotions are central, essential, and welcomed.

In the traditional LSP approach, certified facilitators come from multiple backgrounds, some with therapeutic training, and others, without. Yet, even non-therapeutically trained LSP facilitators conducting the traditional, business-oriented LSP approach quickly discover the methodology evokes affective content. The power of the embodied hand-mind approach, coupled with metaphoric storytelling, elicits emotions, often in unexpected ways. This is part of the power of the methodology as social and storied interactions are exchanged.

As such, in this chapter, we expand upon previously discussed theories and shine a spotlight on two additional theories that emphasise

DOI: 10.4324/9781003260424-11

the social dimension of learning, together with the inextricable link between emotions, meaning-making, and metaphoric storytelling. The two theories are social constructivism as a theory of knowledge (Vygotsky, 1978) and the emotion-focussed "broaden-and-build theory" (Fredrickson, 2001).

Constructivism and social constructivism

The term "constructivism" comes from the Latin *con struere*, which means *to arrange* or *to build* (Guiffrida, 2015, p. 1). This notion of arranging and building is appropriate for a process using interlocking construction bricks. Participants sort, arrange, and build with bricks to share their ideas and stories. The bricks become representational artifacts of participants' thoughts, feelings, and knowledge. Conceptually, the theory of constructivism easily extends into social constructivism by incorporating the influence of others and culture in human growth and development (Vygotsky, 1978). Russian psychologist Lev Vygotsky (1978) argued that individuals are active participants in their own lives and in the creation of their own knowledge (Schreiber & Valle, 2013). In social constructivism, humans use language as the central mechanism for knowledge interpretation, meaning-making, and interaction with others (Akpan et al., 2020; Nathaniel, 2018). Social constructivism theorists also take the view that emotions are central to the human experience, health, and well being (Arciero et al., 2004).

Expanding on this notion, Mahoney (2003) wrote, "Constructivism is a view of humans as active, meaning-making individuals who are afloat on webs of relationships while they are moving along streams of life that relentlessly require new directions and connections" (p. xii). By participating in a socially constructivist learning space, a web of relationships is formed that is actively and continuously dynamic. Participants share ideas with each other in conversational exchanges, typically matched up against prior knowledge or their perceptions about the world, which are highly dependent on the individual's culture.

Therefore, every conversation or encounter between two or more people presents an opportunity for new knowledge to be gained or prior knowledge to be expanded upon. With expanded knowledge, the opportunity exists for new awareness and the potential for growth and change. Consequently, the participatory roles of participants in STP are both a product of and a tool for learning, growth, and change.

Broaden-and-build theory

According to the broaden-and-build theory, positive and negative emotions have distinct and complementary adaptive functions that are associated with cognitive and physiological effects (Fredrickson et al., 2000; Fredrickson, 2001, 2004, 2013). This theory posits that negative emotions narrow one's momentary thought-action repertoire by preparing one to behave in a specific way (often referred to as "fight or flight" responses when feeling angry or afraid). This narrowing of thoughts and actions are necessary to generate quick and decisive action to escape danger (Fredrickson, 2004).

In contrast, various discrete positive emotions (e.g., joy, contentment, interest) broaden one's thought-action repertoire, expanding the range of cognitions and behaviours that come to mind. These broadened mindsets have the capacity to build an individual's physical, intellectual, and social resources, resulting in an openness and ability to engage in higher-order activities (Fredrickson, 2001, 2004). Therefore, experiencing negative emotions reduces the number and range of options available to respond quickly when necessary or under threat, while positive emotions generate or expand the range of options available, resulting in creative, flexible, exploratory, and "out-of-the-box" options or ideas to help solve a problem.

Tugade and Fredrickson's (2007) research explored the temporal aspects of the theory and suggested experiencing positive emotions produces both short-term and longer-term effects. They suggested that, as repeated experiences of positive emotions occur, this broadened mindset has the potential to become habitual. Fredrickson and Losada (2005) state, "Because the broaden-and-build effects of positive affect accumulate and compound over time, positivity can transform individuals for the better, making them healthier, more socially integrated, knowledgeable, effective, and resilient" (p. 679).

Additionally, Tugade and Fredrickson (2007) explored the impact of the theory on physiological responses; specifically, cardiovascular responses. Although both low- and high-resilience individuals experienced equal levels of cardiovascular arousal and a negative experience in response to a stressor, higher trait-resilient individuals with more experience with positive emotions exhibited faster cardiovascular recovery from the negative emotional arousal (Tugade & Fredrickson, 2007). In line with the broaden-and-build theory, the narrowing of thought-action repertoires associated with negative emotions was accompanied by cardiovascular reactivity that prepared the body for specific action. In contrast, positive emotions broadened the thought-action repertoire, which "undid" the lingering cardiovascular after-effects of negative emotions (Fredrickson et al., 2000).

Positive emotions in group work

The role of positive emotions in group work has been studied beyond the broad-and-build theory (Peñalver et al., 2020; van Kleef & Fischer, 2016). Positive emotions have also resulted in group participants' ability to build social supports, gain a sense of membership, enhance communication, experience closeness with others, and in some cases, develop friendships (Catalino & Fredrickson, 2011; Han et al., 2008; Kottman, 2011; Rhee, 2007; Spoor & Kelly, 2004; Wei et al., 2021). Still, other researchers have concluded that positive emotions result in a strengthening of the affiliation function of the group process (van der Schalk et al., 2011; Wei et al., 2021).

Specific to the concept of positive emotions within the LSP context, Wheeler et al. (2020) showed the mere presence of LEGO® bricks were sufficient for the arousal of positive emotions in the participants, ranging from excitement and enthusiasm to curiosity. By using the LEGO® figures metaphorically to represent emotions and thoughts in their stories, participants' emotional vocabulary was evident. This sense of externalisation onto objects helped participants to achieve clarity on their own emotions and thoughts, putting them in a better position to communicate with their team members (Wheeler et al., 2020). Wheeler et al. (2020) also suggested that, as the methodology unfolded, group participants approached more difficult content as collaborators, not adversaries.

Sense-making/meaning-making

One construct embedded across social constructivism and storytelling literature that holds relevance to STP is the concept of sense- or meaning-making (Bietti et al., 2019; Hartog et al., 2020: Thomas et al., 2014; Zittoun & Brinkmann, 2012). Meaning-making is closely related to sense-making, and the two terms are often used interchangeably. For our purposes, we believe sense-making is how we attempt to understand the external world and precedes meaning-making. Meaning-making is how we relate the information from sense-making to our inner world, asking what the situation means personally or in the contexts of our own family, community, organisations, or society. Meaning-making is a process by which individuals interpret the personal impact of events, situations, objects, and conversations alongside previous knowledge and experiences. Within a learning context, both sense- and meaning-making are influenced by cultural views and contexts. (See Chapters 2 and 3 for a discussion on the underlying brain structures which reinforce our separation of sense- and meaning-making.)

One of our favourite ways of making sense and meaning when relating to one another is through sharing stories about ourselves and others (Bruner, 2003; McAdams & Manczak, 2015; Straub, 2005). Several authors have written about how identity is both storied and relational (Freedman & Combs, 2004; Hedtke & Winslade, 2004; White, 2007). The stories we tell ourselves are important, as are the stories we tell others about ourselves and our lives. Likewise, the stories others hear us tell and the stories that they tell about us are equally important because they shape our identities. Stories teach, explain, challenge, inspire, and accordingly, are often filled with metaphors. Metaphors are defined by Lakoff and Johnson (2008) as "understanding of one kind of thing in terms of another" (p. 5) and are an essential element in stimulating new understandings (Jacobs & Heracleous, 2006) (as discussed in Chapters 1, 2, and 5).

Metaphors are ubiquitous in adult communication, enabling adults to convey complex or intangible concepts into a form of expression which otherwise is difficult to describe (Lakoff & Johnson, 2008). Metaphors are especially powerful for accessing the existence of phenomena when situations are unfamiliar, new, or when a phenomenon is unfolding for the individual (Tracy et al., 2006). The role of metaphor in sense- and meaning-making allows participants to explore feelings, assumptions, and behaviours in non-threatening ways and facilitates introspection and self-awareness (Nardon & Hari, 2021). Through metaphor, humans often articulate deeply felt, implicit emotions about their lived experiences that were otherwise obscured and undiscussable. Metaphors can be powerful tools to transfer internal meaning to external objects to further understand a specific situation, topic, and experience, including emotional content (Peabody, 2021).

Metaphoric storytelling

Metaphoric storytelling is the heart and soul of STP. Behind every metaphoric brick model created and the accompanying story, there are often emotionally rich memories and meaning. As therapeutic facilitators, rather than assume we understand the stories of others, we work to co-construct meaning with the participants. Therefore, instead of avoiding or redirecting emotional content, we must be prepared for and are purposeful in facilitating the expression of emotion in the metaphoric storytelling of STP. This aspect truly differentiates STP from the traditional LSP methodology.

While, in the traditional LSP methodology, emotions are certainly present, the basic tenets and etiquette are to question the model and its story, not the person. While keeping the focus on the model and metaphors is also true in STP, the therapeutic facilitator listens closely and carefully for emotional content as participants share their stories. The facilitator then extends the affective components through questions or comments, fully understanding the prominent role of emotions in sense- and meaning-making.

The STP facilitator invites and encourages emotional content to be shared amongst the group members, if it is related to the participants' model and story. Rather than hurry, disregard, or avoid emotional content, in STP, the facilitator allows emotions to serve as the prominent focus, and they are the litmus test for growth and change. Therapeutic facilitators do not downplay or work around emotions that are present during the group experiences; rather, they welcome emotions and are cognisant of how emotions are foundational and intertwined with health, well being, and decision-making.

The interplay of emotions in metaphoric storytelling

Many scholars have written about the interplay of emotions, metaphors, and storytelling (Gibbs et al., 2002; Hammel, 2018; Nadeau, 2006; Snævarr, 2006). The research by Gibbs et al. (2002) suggests that metaphorical language communicates more emotional intensity to listeners than literal language. Additionally, Habermas (2019) has written that emotions are the preferred objects of metaphors (p. 56).

When individuals engage in meaning-making about personal or professional change, they can become vulnerable and show one's own uncertainty or fear (Brown, 2015). Yet, this sharing has the potential to prompt others to feel more comfortable in doing so as well (Brown, 2015). Indeed, when people share their emotions around change, they are also more likely to be able to problem-solve, find collective hope, and brave challenges (Brown, 2015). Taken together, the body of research on metaphoric storytelling shows the integral role of collective emotional expression and how metaphors provide access to that emotional experience, offering paths towards collective healing and well being (Aita et al., 2003).

Therefore, with metaphoric model building, storytelling, and discourse around emotional experiences, the STP facilitator must be skilled in navigating emotional content within the group process. In STP, emotional expression is encouraged, rather than avoided. However, STP is not a therapeutic discipline; rather, it borrows transdisciplinary concepts from storytelling and narrative approaches to engage in the therapeutic process. Therapeutic facilitators who are trained therapists most likely have comfort in a range of skills to explore emotional content; however, if one is not a trained therapist, it is imperative and ethical to practice within the boundaries of your training. We believe that skilled facilitation is complex and sophisticated, requiring facilitators to be prepared and plan for emotional content to enter the socially constructed learning space at any time.

The role of the therapeutic facilitator

Creating the space for emotional-content sharing does not just magically happen. The therapeutic facilitator is the linchpin to mediating and structuring the overall dynamic group process and vital to the overall success of the experience. The skills of the therapeutic facilitator create a fluid and flexible learning space requiring close attention to social dynamics, and facilitators possess the ability to make facilitative responses with sensitivity and respect. The STP facilitator makes intentional choices around the nuances of the group process and pacing and the selection of model-building prompts as well as in creating a relationally safe environment where socially co-constructed learning can occur.

In the book titled *The Culture Code*, Coyle (2018) suggests a metaphoric description of vulnerability in group settings when he writes that vulnerability precedes trust. Coyle (2018) believes leaping into the unknown alongside others causes trust to materialise and form a solid foundation or ground beneath us. Whether you agree with Coyle's temporal sequence or believe trust comes before vulnerability, clearly the therapeutic facilitator plays a significant role in inviting and creating trust and vulnerability. The therapeutic facilitator also has a role in witnessing and holding the relational group process.

"Bearing witness" and "holding the environment" are psychological terms often used in expressive psychotherapies (Pikiewicz, 2013). The terms refer to sharing experiences with others, usually by communicating about traumatic experiences to help process the experience through catharsis and receiving empathy (Pikiewicz, 2013). Although the terms are typically used in trauma treatment, the terms and their meaning can also have relevance in non-trauma contexts. However, many people bear witness daily with others through conversation, writing, or art and not necessarily about traumatic content. While bearing witness is vital in the therapeutic recovery from trauma, we all have our stories to tell, even in the absence of trauma. Sharing ourselves with others opens up a space where there once was none and often allows growth and resilience to prevail. The following quote by Pikiewicz (2013) sums it up nicely:

> Although the tale of human experience is certainly universal, it contains unique elements for each of us, and we continue the art of storytelling, both verbally and nonverbally, each and every day. While some stories are sweeter than others, all long for the benefit and necessity of a witness, for a witness assures us that our stories are heard, contained, and transcend time; for it can be said that one is never truly forgotten when one is shared and carried in the hearts of others.

The psychoanalyst Winnicott (1960) referred to the "holding" environment as the supportive environment that a therapist or group facilitator creates for the client or group members to include nurturing, caring behaviours that result in trust and safety (Winnicott, 1960). Entering a holding environment requires the therapist or facilitator to tolerate uncertainty, complexity, and navigate relational components (Atlas & Aron, 2017; Mitchell, 2000). While STP itself is not therapy, it is not unusual that many individuals have experienced some type of experience that was difficult for them, and we must be aware that information shared may be triggering for some individuals. Facilitators must be prepared to hold a safe space while supporting the individual within a group setting.

In STP, the therapeutic facilitator encourages relationships to strengthen throughout the group experience. Positive relationships include a "pedagogy of connection" with a focus on how the understandings and feelings of connection are uniquely co-created between specific participants in the specific time and place of the group experience

(Hinz et al., 2022). Applying a relationally based view of group conversations presents a mutuality approach that includes both listening and speaking for connection (Hinz et al., 2022).

Cunliffe's (2008) relationally responsive social constructionism stance proposes that "we create our sense of, and meanings about, our social surroundings and ourselves in our conversations and interactions with those around us." This view suggests that the conversational context is one in which people mutually co-create high-quality connections and positive relationships. It is from these perspectives that "being relational" involves listeners being active contributors to conversations in ways uniquely shaped toward the speaker, what is being shared, and the immediate context. These conversations often elicit certain feelings and responses (Stephens & Lyddy, 2016), and it is the complexity of this mutual interactivity that opens up the potential for new ideas and influences that trigger adaptation, learning, and growth (Boyatzis, 2008; Dutton & Heaphy, 2003; Hinz et al., 2022).

When therapeutic facilitators create psychologically relational spaces that focus on mutuality in conversation, participants may experience how being relational with others in their communication elicits a more dynamic understanding of self, other, and group relationships. Relationally based therapeutic facilitators fill a provocative role, as they constantly confirm, stretch, and challenge participants in a careful mix of experiences that honours and enables the individual's personal investment of "me" to also expand to "we" as the group process unfolds. One way that the shift from "me to we" is built into the STP approach is through the application of the LSP shared building.

Shared builds

While the STP process always begins with individual builds, if the opportunity and time allow, the group advances to shared building and group builds. While some STP experiences may stay with only individual LEGO® builds, it is in the shared and group builds that the symmetry of both "me and we" is activated and the therapeutic factors of change brought about through group work become amplified. Moving from "me to we" in a group format has multiple impacts. If the group will continue to meet or work together, then a range of problem-solving issues can be introduced and worked through. If the group is one with no long-term commitment after the group ends, then the momentary validation from group members becomes a place for social input, differing perspectives, and emotional sharing.

Borrowing from LSP, shared models are built by combining individual models into one model, through a process of dialogue, negotiation, and agreement to create shared understanding and consensus around a particular topic (Kristiansen & Rasmussen, 2014). This process occurs by participants integrating parts of their individual models or complete individual models. In the shared-model application, all participants build their individual responses to the building prompt before engaging in the shared model-building process to ensure everybody's voice is heard and that everybody will have something to contribute to the shared model.

A shared model-building process has the purpose of getting as many details and nuances of the group's reflections into the shared model, striving towards capturing the essence of the prompt, which each of the group members can accept and recognise as part of their shared reality. Reaching this type of recognition, again, requires excellent therapeutic facilitation skills, as the process is a lateral transformation from "me to we," allowing for individual thoughts to remain while new communal thoughts emerge.

If time and goals of the group align, the therapeutic facilitator can continue to the next phase of the process, titled "creating a landscape," with a different prompt (Kristiansen & Rasmussen, 2014). In this phase, the goal is to analyse or categorise the collection of individual models, without losing the meaning, while participants look for common patterns and differences. Participants may physically move individual models closer or further away from others on the table space (Kristiansen & Rasmussen, 2014). Again, the therapeutic facilitator asks extending questions, makes observations, notices, and communicates in a way that encourages all to engage in the landscape building and storytelling.

Next, in the following phase of the application, participants engage in making connections. Using LEGO® chains, tubes, hoses, or strings, participants look to identify relationships or points of connection between constructed models. These connections can be flexible or weak or strong but are visually put out on the table, making the relationships observable. The ensuing dialogue typically strengthens group engagement, and it is the responsibility of the therapeutic group facilitator to continuously create, build, and strengthen the psychological safety of the group experience (Dykes, 2018).

As previously mentioned, even in the traditional LSP process, facilitators acknowledge that emotions are quickly shared in the metaphoric stories built with the bricks. This comes as no surprise to STP facilitators, who are targeting therapeutic applications of the traditional model and argue emotions drive learning in social contexts. Emotions serve critical roles in directing our attention, shaping our perceptions, organising our memory, and motivating our active engagement with the learning that occurs around us.

Conclusion

It is increasingly important to build, broaden, and continuously grow our knowledge base about successful interventions. In this chapter, we focussed on moving from a "me," or individual, lens to a "we" perspective, deepening our understanding of the role that emotions play in STP. We explored two additional theories that underpin the group process: social constructivism and the broad-and-build theory and how both social theories can be conceptualised through the role of emotions in learning and group processes.

Emotions are inseparable from human beings and human groups; therefore, as therapeutic facilitators in STP, we must identify and support the emotions that exist in our participants. Emotions are indispensable parts of storytelling, helping with sense- and meaning-making, helping to understand ourselves and others, and identifying opportunities. This central attention to emotions is one of the differentiating factors between the traditional LSP methodology and the STP approach. Listening for emotions, working directly with emotions, and understanding their purpose are all key facilitation skills that create a safe communal space for sharing and growing.

The paradox for facilitators using STP is that there is a defined therapeutic purpose and learning objectives, yet the facilitator must be flexible and comfortable to manage the emotional content that will inevitably arise. If one wants to use the power of metaphors, stories, and bricks to connect and grow in health and well being in a therapeutic context, it is important to acknowledge and respect your own professional boundaries; to seek appropriate feedback and consultation.

The benefits for emotional well being, learning, and decision making are greatly enriched when facilitators and participants welcome emotions into the STP process as essential and intertwined with growth and change experiences for individuals and within social relationships. The shared learning space that holds emotions for the individual and for the group, from "me to we," is dynamic and empowering. In STP, we invite emotions to be part of the engaging and empowering process, and above all else, we honour and respect emotions as core to the essence of being human.

References

Aita, V., McIlvain, H., Susman, J., & Crabtree, B. (2003). Using metaphor as a qualitative analytic approach to understand complexity in primary care research. *Qualitative Health Research*, *13*(10), 1419–1431. https://doi.org/10.1177/1049732303255999

Akpan, V. I., Igwe, U. A., Mpamah, I. B. I., & Okoro, C. O. (2020). Social constructivism: Implications on teaching and learning. *British Journal of Education*, *8*(8), 49–56.

Arciero, G., Gaetano, P., Maselli, P., & Gentili, N. (2004). Identity, personality and emotional regulation. In A. Freeman, M. J. Mahoney, P. Devito, & D. Martin (Eds.), *Cognition and psychotherapy* (2nd ed., pp. 261–272). Springer. www.ipra.it/articoli/english-identity-personality-and-emotional-regulation-2/

Atlas, G., & Aron, L. (2017). *Dramatic dialogue: Contemporary clinical practice* (1st ed.). Routledge. https://doi.org/10.4324/9781315150086

Bietti, L. M., Tilston, O., & Bangerter, A. (2019). Storytelling as adaptive collective sensemaking. *Topics in Cognitive Science*, *11*(4), 710–732. https://doi.org/10.1111/tops.12358

Boyatzis, R. E. (2008). Leadership development from a complexity perspective. *Consulting Psychology Journal: Practice and Research*, *60*(4), 298–313. https://doi.org/10.1037/1065-9293.60.4.298

Brown, B. (2015). *Daring greatly: How the courage to be vulnerable transforms the way we live, love, parent, and lead.* Penguin.

Bruner, J. (2003). *Making stories: Law, literature, life.* Farrar, Straus, and Giroux Publishing.

Catalino, L. I., & Fredrickson, B. L. (2011). A Tuesday in the life of a flourisher: The role of positive emotional reactivity in optimal mental health. *Emotion*, *11*(4), 938–950. https://doi.org/10.1037/a0024889

Coyle, D. (2018). *The culture code.* Bantam Books.

Cunliffe, A. L. (2008). Orientations to social constructionism: Relationally responsive social constructionism and its implications for knowledge and learning. *Management Learning*, *39*(2), 123–139. https://doi.org/10.1177/1350507607087578

Dutton, J., & Heaphy, E. (2003). The power of high-quality connections. In K. Cameron, J. Dutton, & R. E. Quinn (Eds.), *Positive organizational scholarship: Foundations of a new discipline* (pp. 262–278). Berrett-Koehler Publishers.

Dykes, W. W. (2018). *Play well: Constructing creative confidence with LEGO® SERIOUS PLAY®* [Doctoral dissertation, Fielding Graduate University]. www.academia. edu/42964534/Play_Well_Constructing_Creative_Confidence_With_LEGO_ Serious_Play?auto=download

Fredrickson, B. L. (2001). The role of positive emotions in positive psychology: The broaden-and-build theory of positive emotions. *American Psychologist, 56*(3), 218–226. https://doi.org/10.1037/0003-066X.56.3.218

Fredrickson, B. L. (2004). The broaden-and-build theory of positive emotions. *Philosophical Transactions of the Royal Society of London: Series B, Biological Sciences, 359*(1449), 1367–1378. https://doi.org/10.1098/rstb.2004.1512

Fredrickson, B. L. (2013). Positive emotions broaden and build. In P. Devine & A. Plant (Eds.), *Advances in experimental social psychology* (Vol. 47, pp. 1–53). Academic Press. https://doi.org/10.1016/B978-0-12-407236-7.00001-2

Fredrickson, B. L., & Losada, M. (2005). Positive affect and the complex dynamics of human flourishing. *American Psychologist, 60*, 678–686. https://doi. org/10.1037/0003-066X.60.7.678

Fredrickson, B. L., Mancuso, R. A., Branigan, C., & Tugade, M. M. (2000). The undoing effect of positive emotions. *Motivation and Emotion, 24*, 237–258. https://doi. org/10.1023/A:1010796329158

Freedman, J., & Combs, G. (2004). Relational identity in narrative work with couples. In S. Madigan (Ed.), *Therapy from the outside in*. Yaletown Family Therapy.

Gibbs, R. W., Leggitt, J. S., & Turner, E. A. (2002). What's special about figurative language in emotional communication? In S. R. Fussell (Ed.), *The verbal communication of emotions* (pp. 133–158). Psychology Press. https://doi.org/10.4324/ 9781410606341-13

Guiffrida, D. A. (2015). *Constructive clinical supervision in counseling and psychotherapy*. Routledge. https://doi.org/10.4324/9781315890227

Habermas, T. (2019). *Emotion and narrative: Perspectives in autobiographical storytelling*. Cambridge University Press. https://doi.org/10.1017/9781139424615

Hammel, S. (2018). *Handbook of therapeutic storytelling: Stories and metaphors in psychotherapy, child and family therapy, medical treatment, coaching and supervision*. Routledge. https://doi.org/10.4324/9780429461606

Han, J. Y., Shaw, B. R., Hawkins, R. P., Pingree, S., McTavish, F., & Gustafson, D. H. (2008). Expressing positive emotions within online support groups by women with breast cancer. *Journal of Health Psychology, 13*(8), 1002–1007. https://doi. org/10.1177/1359105308097963

Hartog, I., Scherer-Rath, M., Kruizinga, R., Netjes, J., Henriques, J., Nieuwkerk, P., Sprangers, M., & van Laarhoven, H. (2020). Narrative meaning making and integration: Toward a better understanding of the way falling ill influences quality of life. *Journal of Health Psychology, 25*(6), 738–754. https://doi.org/10.1177/ 1359105317731823

Hedtke, L., & Winslade, J. (2004). *Remembering lives: Conversations with the dying and the bereaved*. Routledge.

Hinz, J., Stephens, J. P., & Van Oosten, E. B. (2022). Toward a pedagogy of connection: A critical view of being relational in listening. *Management Learning, 53*(1), 76–97. https://doi.org/10.1177/13505076211047506

Issah, M. (2018). Change leadership: The role of emotional intelligence. *SAGE Open, 8*(3), 215824401880091. https://doi.org/10.1177/2158244018800910

Jacobs, C. D., & Heracleous, L. T. (2006). Constructing shared understanding: The role of embodied metaphors in organization development. *The Journal of Applied Behavioral Science, 42*(2), 207–226. https://doi.org/10.1177/0021886305284895

Kottman, T. (2011). *Play therapy: Basics and beyond*. American Counseling Association.

Kristiansen, P., & Rasmussen, R. (2014). *Building a better business using the LEGO® SERIOUS PLAY® method*. John Wiley & Sons.

Lakoff, G., & Johnson, M. (2008). *Metaphors we live by*. University of Chicago Press.

Mahoney, M. J. (2003). *Constructive psychotherapy: Theory and practice*. Guilford Press.

McAdams, D. P., & Manczak, E. (2015). Personality and the life story. In M. Mikulincer, P. R. Shaver, M. L. Cooper, & R. J. Larsen (Eds.), *APA handbook of personality and social psychology: Vol. 4. Personality processes and individual differences* (pp. 425–446). American Psychological Association. https://doi.org/10.1037/14343-019

Mitchell, S. A. (2000). *Relationality: From attachment to intersubjectivity*. Analytic Press.

Nadeau, J. W. (2006). Metaphorically speaking: The use of metaphors in grief therapy. *Illness, Crisis & Loss, 14*(3), 201–221. https://doi.org/10.1177/10541373060 1400301

Nardon, L., & Hari, A. (2021). Sensemaking through metaphors: The role of imaginative metaphor elicitation in constructing new understandings. *International Journal of Qualitative Methods, 20*, 160940692110195. https://doi.org/10.1177/16094069211019589

Nathaniel, K. A. (2018). Readiness for practice in social work through a constructionist lens. *Field Educator: Simmons School of Social Work, 8*(2), 1–21.

Peabody, M. A. (2021). Building understanding in parent consultation: Brick by brick. *Play Therapy, 16*(1), 4–7.

Peñalver, J., Salanova, M., & Martínez, I. M. (2020). Group positive affect and beyond: An integrative review and future research agenda. *International Journal of Environmental Research and Public Health, 17*(20), 7499. https://doi.org/10.3390/ijerph17207499

Pikiewicz, K. (2013). The power and strength of bearing witness. *Psychology Today*. www.psychologytoday.com/us/blog/meaningful-you/201312/the-power-and-strength-bearing-witness

Rhee, S.-Y. (2007). Group emotions and group outcomes: The role of group-member interactions. In E. A. Mannix, M. A. Neale, & C. P. Anderson (Eds.), *Affect and groups* (Vol. 10, pp. 65–95). Emerald Group Publishing Limited. https://doi.org/10.1016/S1534-0856(07)10004-9

Schreiber, L. M., & Valle, B. E. (2013). Social constructivist teaching strategies in the small group classroom. *Small Group Research, 44*(4), 395–411. https://doi.org/10.1177/1046496413488422

Seijts, G., & O'Farrell, G. (2003). Engage the heart: Appealing to the emotions facilitates change. *Ivey Business Journal Online*, 1–6.

Snævarr, S. (2006). Emoting and metaphoring: The metaphoric structure of emotions. *Sats – Nordic Journal of Philosophy, 7*(1). https://doi.org/10.1515/SATS.2006.175

Spoor, J. R., & Kelly, J. R. (2004). The evolutionary significance of affect in groups: Communication and group bonding. *Group Processes & Intergroup Relations, 7*(4), 398–412. https://doi.org/10.1177/1368430204046145

Stephens, J. P., & Lyddy, C. J. (2016). Operationalizing heedful interrelating: How attending, responding, and feeling comprise coordinating and predict performance in self-managing teams. *Frontiers in Psychology, 7.* www.frontiersin.org/articles/10.3389/fpsyg.2016.00362

Straub, J. (2005). Telling stories, making history: Toward a narrative psychology of the historical construction of meaning. In J. Straub (Ed.), *Narration, identity, and historical consciousness* (pp. 44–98). Berghahn Books.

Thomas, A., Menon, A., Boruff, J., Rodriguez, A. M., & Ahmed, S. (2014). Applications of social constructivist learning theories in knowledge translation for healthcare professionals: A scoping review. *Implementation Science, 9*(1), 54. https://doi.org/10.1186/1748-5908-9-54

Tracy, S. J., Lutgen-Sandvik, P., & Alberts, J. K. (2006). Nightmares, demons, and slaves: Exploring the painful metaphors of workplace bullying. *Management Communication Quarterly, 20*(2), 148–185. https://doi.org/10.1177/0893318906291980

Tugade, M. M., & Fredrickson, B. L. (2007). Regulation of positive emotions: Emotion regulation strategies that promote resilience. *Journal of Happiness Studies, 8*(3), 311–333. https://doi.org/10.1007/s10902-006-9015-4

Turesky, E., & Peabody, M. A. (2018). University identity change through a psychological sense of community framework: A case study of the ELIMAR model. *International Journal of Leadership and Change, 6*(1), 43–54.

van der Schalk, J., Fischer, A., Doosje, B., Wigboldus, D., Hawk, S., Rotteveel, M., & Hess, U. (2011). Convergent and divergent responses to emotional displays of ingroup and outgroup. *Emotion, 11*(2), 286–298. https://doi.org/10.1037/a0022582

van Kleef, G. A., & Fischer, A. H. (2016). Emotional collectives: How groups shape emotions and emotions shape groups. *Cognition and Emotion, 30*(1), 3–19. https://doi.org/10.1080/02699931.2015.1081349

Vygotsky, L. S. (1978). *Mind in society: Development of higher psychological processes* (M. Cole & V. John-Steiner, Trans.). Harvard University Press.

Watkins, D., Earnhardt, M., Pittenger, L., Roberts, R., Rietsema, K., & Cosman-Ross, J. (2017). Thriving in complexity: A framework for leadership education. *Journal of Leadership Education, 16*(4), 148–163. https://doi.org/10.12806/V16/I4/T4

Wei, M., Wang, L., & Kivlighan, D. M. (2021). Group counseling change process: An adaptive spiral among positive emotions, positive relations, and emotional cultivation/regulation. *Journal of Counseling Psychology, 68*(6), 730–745. https://doi.org/10.1037/cou0000550

Wheeler, S., Passmore, J., & Gold, R. (2020). All to play for: LEGO® SERIOUS PLAY® and its impact on team cohesion, collaboration and psychological safety in organisational settings using a coaching approach. *Journal of Work-Applied Management, 12*(2), 141–157. https://doi.org/10.1108/JWAM-03-2020-0011

White, M. (2007). *Maps of narrative practice* (pp. x, 304). W. W. Norton & Company.

Winnicott, D. (1960). The theory of the parent-child relationship. *International Journal of Psychoanalysis, 41*, 585–595.

Zittoun, T., & Brinkmann, S. (2012). Learning as meaning making. In N. M. Seel (Ed.), *Encyclopedia of the sciences of learning* (pp. 1809–1811). Springer US. https://doi.org/10.1007/978-1-4419-1428-6_1851

Chapter 11

Putting it into play

Practical applications and case studies

Mary Anne Peabody, Alec Hamilton, and Kristen Klassen

This is a much less academic chapter and harkens back to our personal experiences of developing our ideas and using LEGO® therapeutically – i.e., Seriously Therapeutic Play with LEGO® (STP). We provided snapshots of a range of "cases" – from individual therapy to group therapy (both virtual and in-person) to families and parent consultations to supervision and current implementations of the methodology – are detailed. Quotes and pictorial examples from our work with participants express not only the 3-D nature of the bricks but also the dynamism of the approach, which allows us to see what "jumps out," "what's now there that wasn't there before," and "what your hands have expressed that your words didn't." It is not our aim to demonstrate the full depth of the STP process here; we will leave that for the next book.

You will find seven case studies presented in this chapter. We have tried to make the structure the same across each case study. We start with the context of the situation. Follow this with any presenting challenges. We then briefly articulate the STP process we used. Finally, we discuss the participant and facilitator insights that arose from the process. The models presented in the images are reconstructions of participants' builds with slight modifications to protect the identity of the participants.

DOI: 10.4324/9781003260424-12

1. School-age child: "Ash" – the value of experiments.
2. Adolescent: "Andy" – exploring social relationships.
3. Adult: "Stacy" – untying internal tangles.
4. Clinical supervision: the privilege of being a parent.
5. Parent group: military non-deployed parent psychoeducation group.
6. Virtual group: building through a screen.
7. Higher education: playful teaching and learning.

Case study #1: School-age child: "Ash" – the value of experiments

As many clinicians know, LEGO® and children are a natural fit. It turns out this applies to the STP approach too! Our first case study details the use of the method with an elementary school child.

Context

Ash was 5 years old at the time of the events and in their first year of school. Ash had been having trouble maintaining friendships and was getting into trouble for some behaviour the teacher had described as impulsive. The class teacher believes Ash is intelligent, quick-witted, a good reader, and academically capable. The teacher thinks they are managing some issues with classroom behaviour. The teacher has met with Ash's parents several times and, in term 3 (just after the mid-year break), placed Ash on a behaviour plan. The plan involved a traditional reward chart that rates Ash's behaviour during break times: a tick for good behaviour and a cross for poor behaviour. The goal was for Ash to obtain three out of four positive ticks each day and receive a reward from either their parents or the teacher. If Ash received 12 ticks, then they could obtain a bonus reward.

Challenge

The main challenge was that the reward chart didn't modify Ash's behaviour. There was a slight decrease in peer-related issues, but this arose from Ash choosing to play alone. Ash then started to get into "more serious" trouble for the things they were doing. The first incident that escalated the situation was when Ash went into the toilets. They rolled up the toilet paper, put it in the sink, and ran the water tap. Ash then left the room. As a result, the floor became flooded, which needed to be mopped up by a staff member. The view held by the teacher and administration was that Ash was being naughty and, at some level, was being deliberate in his negative behaviour. The teacher placed Ash on a more stringent behaviour plan and sent him to "behaviour chat," which involves a reflection process with a senior member of staff where Ash is asked to reflect on their behaviour and how they might repair the problem. The incident that called for my more direct involvement occurred 2 months after the first bathroom incident, when Ash, again, flooded the bathroom. They had picked some berries from the garden area, squashed them into a paste, and then placed them in the toilet, followed by a lot of paper.

Once caught, Ash said they knew they were in trouble and their parents would be angry. They couldn't or wouldn't talk to the administration staff member about the incident and just sat and cried. I had a chance to chat with Ash a day or so later.

Process

Ash and I talked for a while about things they liked doing and some of the good things about school. I then told Ash I was interested in what happened the other day with the toilet. Ash didn't want to talk about it. I asked if they would like to play with some LEGO®. I gave them a kit, and they started to build quietly. I eventually asked Ash if they could build what happened with the toilet. Ash agreed and began to build quite a complex model. Then we chatted about the model (Figure 11.1):

Can you point to each part and tell me what each part is?

- This is me.
- This is the toilet, and I'm blocking the toilet or something, but I can't remember. And this is my thinking.
- I'm thinking that it's gonna go blast.

So, you wanted to see if the toilet would "go blast" if you filled it with things and flushed it?
Yep. I wanted to see it explode and water shoot up. (Ash was smiling and laughing in a cheeky, wicked way, pointing to their face in the model.)

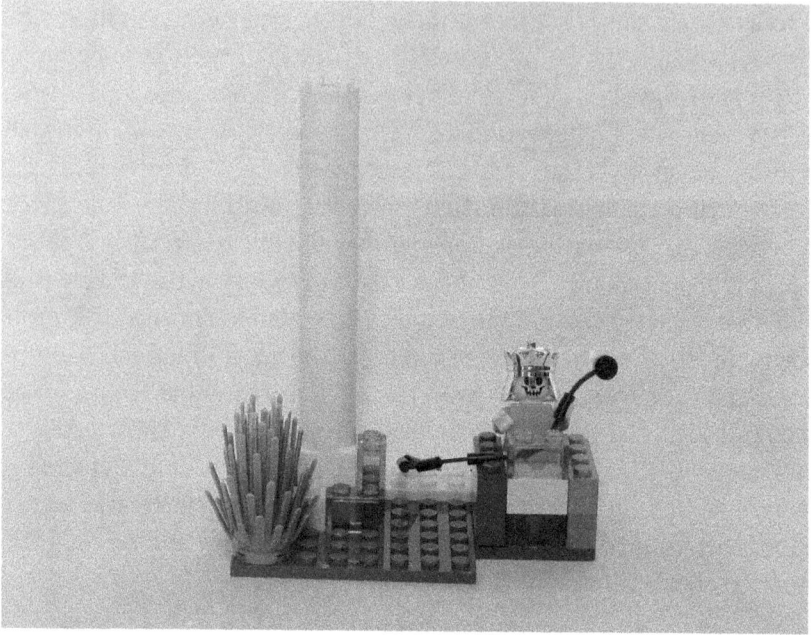

Figure 11.1 *The exploding toilet experiment.*

It seems like a bit of a science experiment. Do you like finding out
how things work?

Yep, I do lots of experiments.

Insights

Participant

Ash was, for the first time, able to tell the story from his perspective – not
from the perspective of someone getting in trouble. They wanted to see
it explode. It hadn't happened the first time with the sink, so I believe
Ash thought they would try it again with more active ingredients. They
weren't trying to be naughty, but rather, experimenting with the toilet.
We talked about how they felt when they were in trouble. Ash said they
felt sorry when the teachers spoke to them. But they didn't think to stop
while they were doing things.

Facilitator

When we chatted at the beginning of the session, Ash seemed to try to
tell me what they thought I wanted them to say – trying to stay out of

trouble. As Ash started to build the LEGO® model, they were focussed on the model; their attention was away from me. Ash became more animated and played out the role of the exploding toilet with sound effects. I could see the excitement and joy of the "scientist" working out their experiment and their disappointment that it hadn't exploded as they had hoped. The LEGO® build process allowed me to implement a different strategy for break times. We now focussed on supporting the scientist, helping him engage with his peers and productively use his curiosity and intelligence rather than focusing on just staying out of trouble. The initial process had not unearthed Ash's motivation but simply brought out his defensive response to being in trouble. I think this was the first time Ash had been heard and seen as a scientist, and I think Ash felt good about this view of them.

Case study #2: Adolescent: "Andy" – exploring social relationships

Our second case study focuses on the adolescent experience. This case example was chosen to illustrate how STP assists in promoting the clients' and the clinicians' shared understanding of a situation.

Context

How STP assists in promoting the clients – and my shared understanding of a situation – is illustrated in the following case example. A core aspect of working with children and adolescents in a school situation is helping them manage their peer relationships. When clients struggle with their peer relationships, I often ask them to describe their friendship group in words, draw a sociogram diagram, or build a LEGO® model. To illustrate the point, I've presented an amalgam of several student interactions with one student's story at the core of the narrative. The names, pronouns, and specific relationships have been changed to de-identify the student, but the basic story remains. The model replicates the student's model; the description and graphics were constructed from that narrative. I generally do not ask the student to do all three aspects but may use the different strategies at various times throughout the sessions with the student. Information in brackets is provided for clarity and is not part of the narrative.

Challenge

The specific friendship group includes seven students who are all 15 or 16 years old. The year-level coordinator (YLC) reports that they seem age-appropriate in their social and emotional development. There are no academic, emotional, or behavioural issues of which the YLC is aware. However, they are concerned as some of Andy's teachers have reported that "Andy seems withdrawn at the moment." Andy's grades haven't been too affected, but Andy doesn't seem to be the same person the teachers met in term 1. There are no reports of issues at home.

This is Andy's narrative after the "get to know each other" phase of the session.

- I'm in a group of about seven students. Me, Paul, Sarah, Brian, Harry, Matilda, and Jane. I'm feeling pretty sad at the moment. My friendship group is just falling apart, and I feel really out of it.
- Paul and I have most of their classes together.
- Harry is in Andy's class; Brian is in Sarah's class.
- Paul and Sarah have been friends for some time.
- Matilda is new to the school and is in Jane's class.
- None of us are "partnered up," but we have been hanging out since the beginning of the year. (It is currently halfway through the school year.)
- Some of us play sport together outside of school.

Process
I asked Andy to verbally explain the current situation

"I'm friendly with Paul, they are my best friend, but Paul's best friend is Sarah. My other friends are Jane, Brian, Matilda and Harry. We go out a lot together, but I often feel left out. Brian and Harry usually stick together, leaving Jane, Matilda and me sitting with Paul and Sarah. Then Sarah and Paul go off, leaving me with the other two, chatting, and I feel out of it. This happens most days."

I asked Andy to draw the current situation

The sociogram system I use involves having the young person place their name in the middle of a sheet of paper (Figure 11.2). Then ask them to imagine that there are concentric rings around themselves with the circle

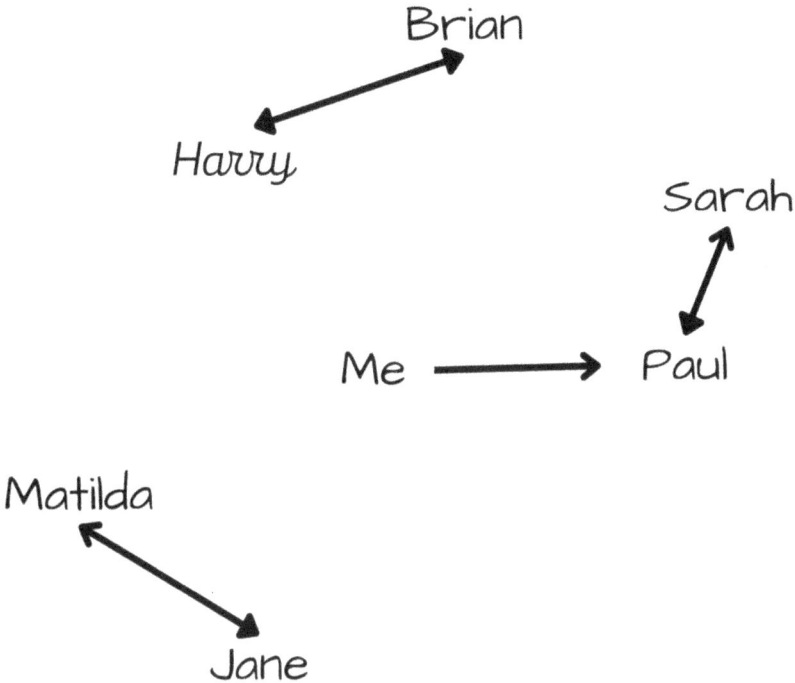

Figure 11.2 *Andy's sociogram.*

nearer their dot/name containing their best friends and those less "best-friend" are placed further out from the centre. Starting with their best friend, they move out from the centre and try to include all their friends in the group. The coloured lines are included after the names have been placed on the page. Finally, arrows are added to indicate the direction of the friendship. The direction of the arrows generally shows who are best friends with whom.

Andy's sociogram

- I'm in the centre.
- Paul goes here.
- Then Sarah, who is further away.
- Then Harry, Matilda, and Jane, who are like Paul but a bit further away.
- I don't really know Brian, but they are nice.

Insight – Andy's

- I see now that there are three separate pairs and me.
- I'm only focussed on Paul, and no one is focussed on me.

Andy and I could see the direction of emotional energy flowing within the relationships. They then noticed their isolation.

I asked Andy to build the current situation (Figure 11.3)

Andy's LEGO® build

- This is me (with the blue helmet), and this is my best friend, Paul (with the crown), and this is their best friend, Sarah (long hair).
- We are all friends with Brian, Harry, Matilda, and Jane. Brian and Harry and there (white squares), and Matilda and Jane are there (yellow squares).
- We often all spend time together during breaks and sit around together.

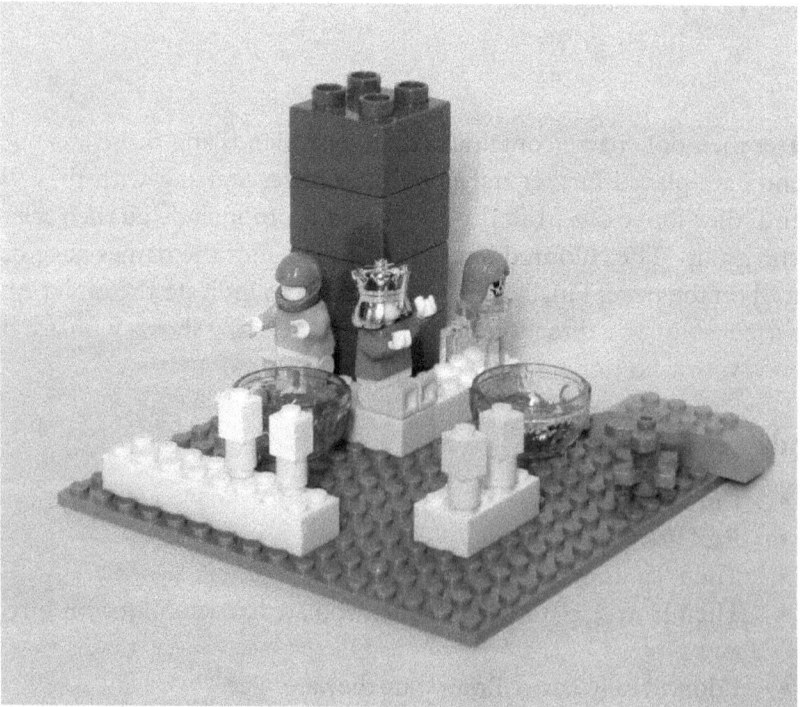

Figure 11.3 *Andy's LEGO® model of the peer group.*

Insight – Andy's

- I see now that there are three separate pairs and me. I'm only focussed on Paul, and no one is focussed on me.
- Paul and Sarah are in this corner with me on the edge. They're at the centre of my circle. Well, mainly Paul; Sarah is out of my circle, really.
- When Paul and Sarah are talking, I'm always left out. Matilda and Jane talk to each other; they're over there. Brian and Harry are talking to each other; they are over here. But I'm left out.
- This is where I want to be (pointing to the space in front of Sarah); that's where all the fun is. That's where the gold is in the garden, but I'm around the corner.
- It's funny I hadn't really noticed how the big, white bricks are blocking me from all the fun. I really am stuck out here on the edge. That orange brick almost has me sliding out of the picture.
- I really do feel like I'm stuck, now that I see the helmet on my own head! I can't see much at all. Actually, I just noticed that my eyes are totally covered; you can't see them! And my little cup is empty of gold.
- The other thing I notice is that I was deliberate in the crown being on Paul's head because he's everyone's favourite.
- Sarah has everything in front of her: the garden, gold, and long, blonde hair. I enjoyed making her "skeleton face."

Insight – facilitator

The depth of the build provides an opportunity for Andy to reflect on things in much greater detail; noticing their own eyes and how they represent Sarah are great examples. The insights allow us to talk about emotional content and how we might move forward in either building the relationships or shifting them in a different direction. It illustrates to me their level of emotion and how they feel physically and emotionally.

Case study #3: Adult: "Stacy" – untying internal tangles

Charles Schaefer (2003) argues that, for adults, play is essential to fostering adaptive behaviours, role rehearsal, and mind-body integration. However, as any play therapist knows, engaging adults to play can be challenging, particularly in a therapeutic context. This case study was chosen to illustrate

STP's power in fully engaging adult participants in an individual therapy setting. Again, identifying details have been changed, and not all meanings in the model have been presented to protect the participant.

Context

Work with "Stacy" began in the spring of 2021. As an adolescent, she was a survivor of an alcoholic parent and a high-conflict divorce. As a young adult, she subsequently had a traumatic and high-conflict relationship of her own. Prior to her arrival in the playroom, she had been working with a therapist for several years and had done significant work repairing her relationship with her non-alcoholic parent. Additionally, she was in a stable and supportive relationship with her current partner and was highly successful in her career. However, she had begun feeling that her therapeutic journey had stagnated. She described herself as being stuck between an old version of herself and a "new, higher version" of herself that she could recognise but could not become.

Challenge

Her primary challenge was severe sociotropy and a compulsion to please others or meet social norms at the expense of her own needs. This pattern was evident in her history of engaging in workplace and social situations which were traditionally male-dominated and presented significant opportunities not only for conflict but also for her to be criticised, rejected, and demeaned. She frequently sacrificed her own needs, such as eating healthy and regular meals, sleeping enough, and exercising regularly, in favour of meeting and exceeding others' expectations. This propensity for people-pleasing was further challenged by the fact that Stacy actively worked to disconnect from her emotional self; she described herself as unfeeling and was frequently unaware of her own emotional state.

Process

LEGO® was introduced in our second session together, and the final model unfolded from three main questions. Stacy was first asked to build a model to represent her internal experience – the parts she did not allow others to see (Figure 11.4). The first part of the model emerged with the tan pieces representing the walls she put up around herself and the skeleton face representing the negative self-image and self-judgement.

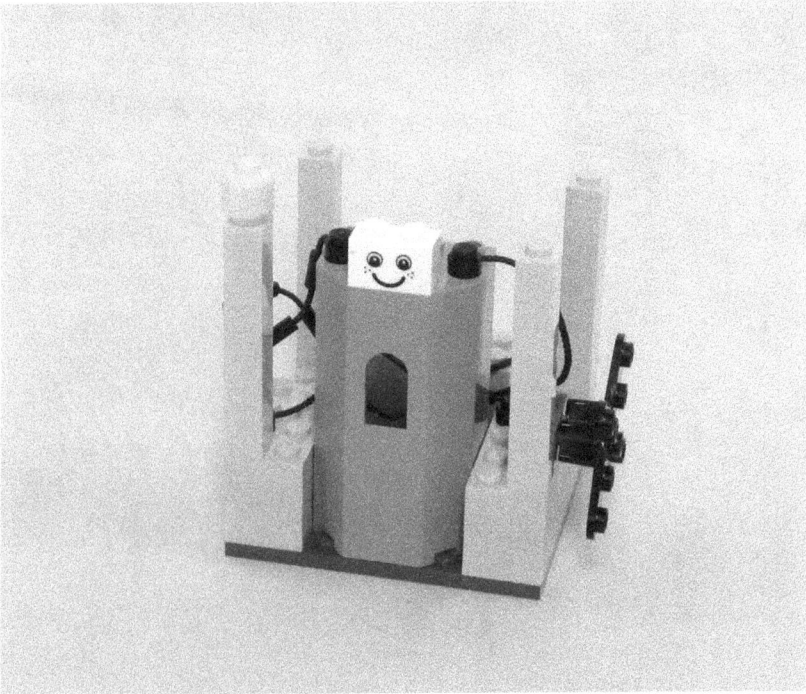

Figure 11.4 *The view of Stacy from the outside; what others are permitted to see.*

A single yellow brick with a smiling face atop the model represented what she showed to the outside world. The black cords wrapped around the core of the model represented the constant indecision she felt concerning how to move forward in her life.

In the discussion of the meaning of the black cords, a second component to her model emerged; a crown was placed on top of a large, white pillar that was inaccessible from all angles (unreachable by stairs, ladder, extension from her internal self, or from the ground; Figure 11.5). She described this component as her true self and her true potential. Even she could not figure out how to reach the golden crown.

After completing and discussing the first two models, Stacy was asked if she could build a model of what she would like her internal experience to be (regardless of whether it was seen or unseen). In response, she built the model on the far right of the following image, indicating an individual "that was at peace with themselves" (Figure 11.6). The window and windshield represented a clarity of perspective in reference to the past and toward the future. The blue piece underlying them represented a

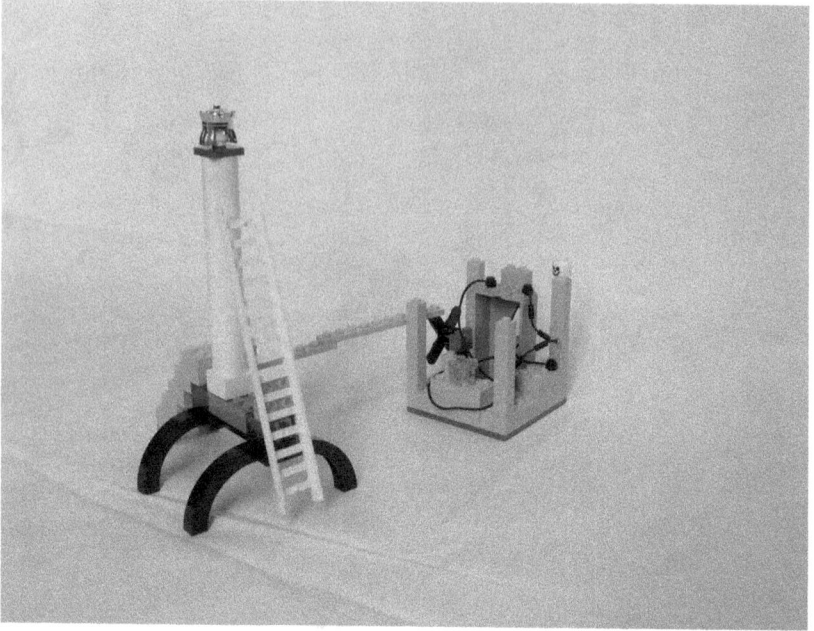

Figure 11.5 *The reverse angle of the previous model with an additional component – the "unreachable crown."*

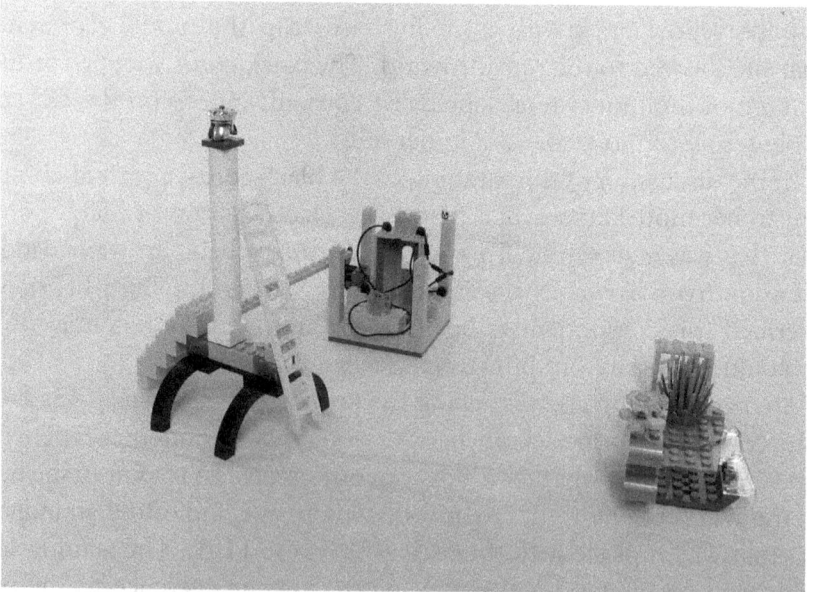

Figure 11.6 *A model in contrast to the previous two, using blue, green, and transparent bricks and windows to represent clarity, peace, beauty, and growth.*

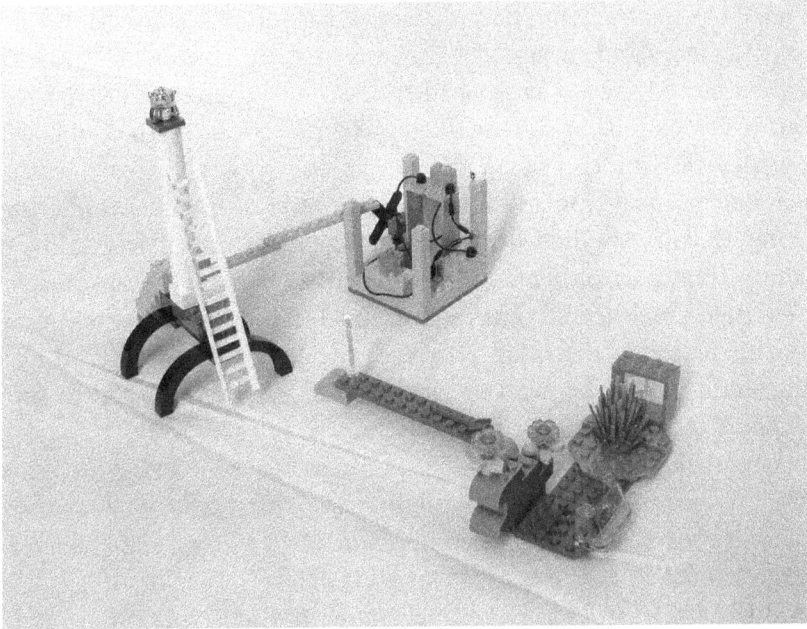

Figure 11.7 *All four models, shown together with a literal bridge linking the models.*

direct and open path between the past and future, and the green and flowers were metaphors for growth, renewal, and an appreciation of the beauty in her life.

Finally, Stacy was asked if she could build a model of what might be the missing piece or pieces between the current state and the ideal state or why she believes this ideal state is so unattainable (Figure 11.7). Her final model placed between the two was a literal bridge with a shovel to denote hard work and a magic wand to indicate some magic or unknown, ethereal force. She placed the final model between the two states of herself. This final model, in the simplicity of the build, in the limited colours and pieces used, and in the description of the meaning, was in stark contrast to the previous three models. This final model took Stacy significantly longer to build than either the current state or the ideal state model, and she was less able to answer questions about this model.

Insights

Participant

As Stacy built her first model, she was initially hesitant to touch the pieces. However, as she began building, the story began to flow easily;

she talked as she built and became almost run-on in her attempt to share all of the pieces and meanings. This was in sharp contrast to the halted and interrupted speech as she had tried to talk about her experience(s) in our previous session. When asked questions about the model or what she built, she would pick up the model and look at it from different angles before answering and acknowledging the components of her story or meaning that she had not seen before or did not intentionally give meaning to as part of her build. At the conclusion of the session, Stacy commented that she had never felt so much freedom in sharing her perspective; she felt that working through the LEGO® had allowed her to (temporarily) drop the need to meet others' expectations and to simply see herself. She commented that she felt truly seen and yet could not understand that experience, as we rarely made eye-contact within the session. When asked what she might take with her from the session, she came back to the second component of her first build (which had emerged without any specific prompting from the facilitator) and discussed the role it might have in her life with a sense of confidence and hope. In subsequent sessions, she frequently returned to the metaphor and story of her "unreachable crown."

Facilitator

As Stacy built the metaphor, which became known as the unreachable crown, I could see her demeanour and affect change; her body posture relaxed, her eyes lit up, and her voice fell in pitch. There was a sense of increased engagement for her and a realisation that her capacity was greater than even she had previously acknowledged. I felt I was witness to an experience of mind-body integration.

My second key insight was recognising that Stacy was not distressed by the final build result. The contrast between the ease with which Stacy built and discussed her first model and her struggle to build and share the final model representing the "how" was stark to me as a facilitator, yet she did not even comment on that model. When I reflected on this session and the meaning of this dissonance (both in terms of ease/unease with which Stacy built and the relative importance we both placed on this), I considered several potential reasons for this progression; was my final question unclear or perhaps too difficult? Did she not hold the answer to this question, either in conscious or unconscious knowledge? Was there insufficient scaffolding or support to reach this final question? Or was she simply tired, exhausted, and overwhelmed by the cognitive or emotional load presented by the session thus far? The number and range of possible reasons for this outcome highlighted for me a key tenet of my therapeutic approach; the client is the expert in their own life and innately knows what they need to heal, and the therapist only needs to provide the conditions for this healing to occur and respectfully follow the client's lead.

Case study #4: Clinical supervision: the privilege of being a parent

As a play therapy supervisor, I have the honour and responsibility to support therapists-in-training through clinical supervision. Clinical supervision has been rightly recognised as one of the key signature pedagogies of counselling and other mental health disciplines (Watkins, 2020). In clinical supervision, play therapists at all stages of development are offered a psychologically safe relationship for sharing struggles, successes, ethical dilemmas, and the numerous wonderments surrounding difficult child and family cases. This case was chosen to detail the role of STP in the supervision relationship.

Context

Given play therapists who work with children also work with their parents, the role of parent engagement is a common topic brought to clinical supervision. There is ample evidence in child therapy generally, and play therapy specifically, that parent involvement and engagement greatly increase the success of treatment (Dowell & Ogles, 2010; Friedberg & McClure, 2015; Lin & Bratton, 2015). While child therapy can be successful without active parent/caregiver engagement, the treatment outcome is typically limiting; therefore, the best practice in child therapy for most clinicians is to provide some level of parent involvement in the treatment approach.

Challenge

The following case example involves one of my supervisees, who continually brought up parent engagement difficulties in her practice. Upon my invitation to explore this more deeply using STP, she was more than willing, as she felt quite frustrated and confused and felt a growing sense of self-doubt was emerging. Using the power of STP as a tool of self-expression, I wanted to tap into her unconscious thoughts and feelings surrounding this identified notion of self-doubt. I intentionally planned to titrate the intensity of the STP prompts, realising that we would most likely need more than one session to build, share, go away, and return to the meaning presented in the STP process.

Process

Prior to using STP, she used the following words to describe a specific parent: *This parent doesn't realise what a privilege it is to be a parent.* I wanted to understand this statement more fully, so I asked her to: *Build a model that expresses what is meant by "the privilege of being a parent."* She crafted a model that placed a small minifigure in the middle of the base plate and several adult minifigures towering over the smaller figure (Figure 11.8). Then she placed other minifigures on the edge of the baseplate, some facing inward and some facing outward. As she shared her story, she spoke about how not everyone who wants to be a parent can be and that parenting was a privilege – a gift that shouldn't be taken lightly. She described that being a parent "should mean" active

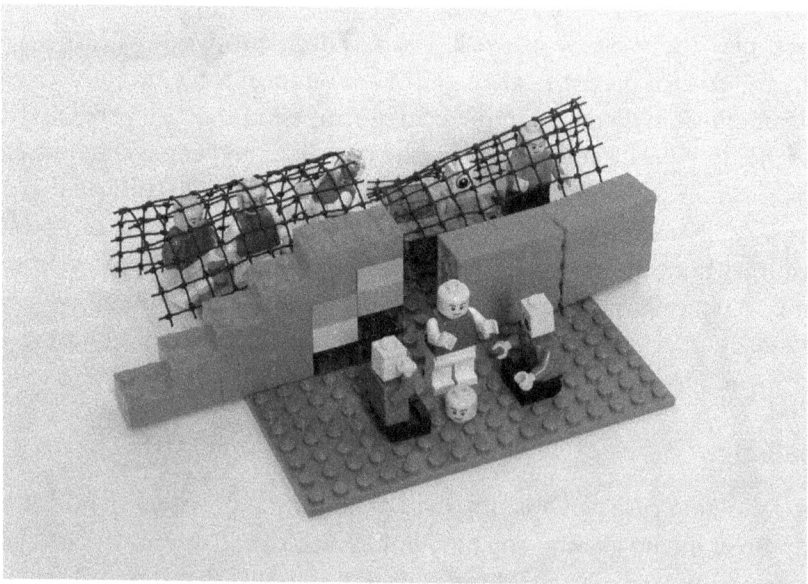

Figure 11.8 *A model showing a small minifigure in the middle of the base plate and several adult minifigures towering over the smaller figure. Minifigures representing parents behind tall brick walls with their hands reaching up with nets over them holding them down.*

involvement, pointing out the proximity dimension of the bricks and how she positioned the minifigures either leaning towards or away from the smaller figure. She described the outwardly facing minifigures on the edge as representations of distant or disengaged parents, and she even removed a couple from the baseplate and placed them further away on the tabletop.

Next, I wanted to have her focus on a model and story around her perceptions of the emotions parents may experience as they bring their children into therapy. The prompt was to *build a model that represented the emotions of some of the parents that she was feeling "stuck" with.* Her model included minifigures representing parents behind tall brick walls; minifigure parents with their hands reaching up while she placed nets over them, holding them down; and minifigures under a pile of bricks. She described her awareness of parental feelings of helplessness in this unfamiliar experience. With permission, we took photographs of the builds. I was especially cognizant of the interconnected building elements of height, walls, and positioning, highlighting the emotional language she used when describing her LEGO® models (Brown & Collins, 2018).

The following week in supervision, I started the session by bringing us back to where we ended by sharing the pictures. In this session, I offered prompts that would now ask her to personalise her own feelings and experiences. Once again, using her own words, I asked her to *build a model that represented her emotions around parent work.* As she built the feelings model, she included frustration, confusion, helplessness, and anger. The anger came as she talked about feeling so helpless to get parents to understand how valuable they were to the therapeutic outcome. She placed a minifigure symbolising herself on the edge of the baseplate, very similar to how she had placed parents in her second model in the previous week.

I was fully aware that we were in the realm of transference, countertransference, and parallel process, which are common phenomena in therapeutic work and certainly appropriate for exploration in clinical supervision. Next, I asked her to *build a model about a time in her past, either personally or professionally, when she experienced her own parental helplessness.*

She carefully built the Newborn Intensive Care Unit (NICU) and placed a tiny brick inside a cradle-shaped LEGO® brick (Figure 11.9). She then attached multiple hoses to the tiny brick and placed numerous

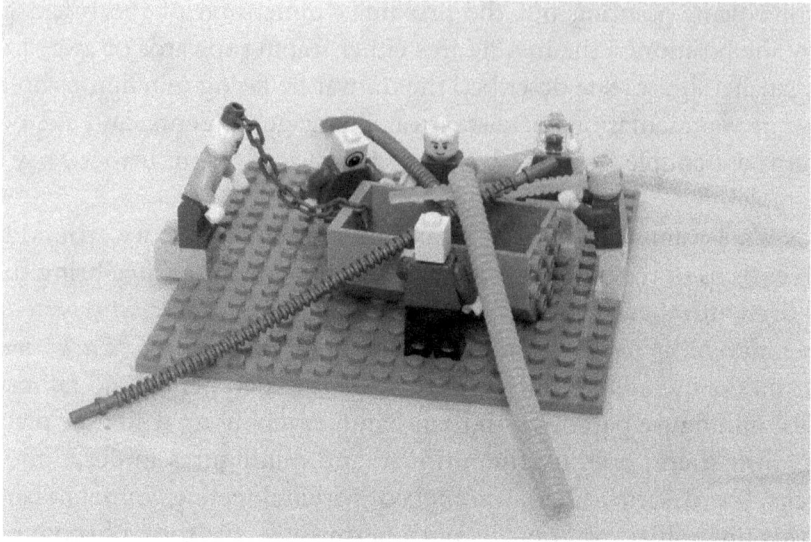

Figure 11.9 *A model representing NICU, with a tiny brick inside a cradle shaped LEGO® brick (representing her son). Multiple hoses run to the tiny brick, and numerous minifigures are all around the cradle. A brick was placed to represent herself on the edge of the base plate, bent over.*

minifigures all around the cradle. She placed a brick on a bent-over mini-figure (herself), placing it on the edge of the base plate. She shared that the tiny brick inside a rectangle brick represented her son inside the incubator. She connected back to her own traumatic memories of being so helpless as a new mother with her newborn son in the NICU. She had felt disconnected in what she had envisioned and dreamed was going to be the "happiest moment of her life." As a therapist-in-training, she had cognitive knowledge around the importance of early attachment and relationships, and she expressed fear that the NICU experience would impair their attachment and recalled how scared, uncertain, and powerless she felt. She shared she paradoxically felt grateful for the full team of health-care professionals working to keep her son alive while also resenting the time, experiences of touch, and the skills they possessed with ease and confidence. The entire experience was very unfamiliar to her as a first-time mother, and her coping mechanisms to deal with all her deep emotions became numbing and slightly detached from all that was happening.

Given our supervision was occurring almost a year and a half after the NICU experience, she wondered if the depth of that traumatic experience might be playing out in the reactions and feelings she was having with the parents of her child clients. We brought the picture of the model she had built about parental feelings around bringing a child to therapy and looked at it together. We discussed the parallel process of how her NICU experience held many of the same emotions that her parents were experiencing. We began to explore how the NICU experience could be spilling over into her clinical treatment responses with parents. Together, we recreated the model, and then, using connecting material from the LSP materials, I asked her to use tubes, connector rods, links, and chains to show the intensity of the connection or a lack of connection.

Insights for the supervisee

She was able to use the bricks to connect her own helplessness of the NICU experience to some of the self-doubt she was feeling around her parental clinical work. She spoke about those early days of attachment uncertainty and wondered if the range of emotions was similar for the parents who sought treatment for their children. She remembered wanting to be involved yet needing to cope by numbing and becoming slightly detached. We explored how these feelings or coping strategies might manifest in what appeared as parental apathy, disconnection, or disengagement. Perhaps the parents in her practice were using this as a protective coping skill. We explored that perhaps parents might view her as the "expert" with skills they did not possess and might experience similar dichotomous feelings of gratefulness and resentfulness. This insight using the bricks provided the emotional distance to create difficult memories and the externalisation necessary to see how the "parent role" was not necessarily resistance but rather something to explore more fully. We continued to explore parental issues and therapeutic use of self in parent consultation to ensure her own feelings of countertransference did not impact the professional space she held with her clients' parents. Eventually, she decided to seek her own therapy to cope with on-going anxiety around her own parenting and to ensure that her own feelings did not impact her professional work.

Insight for the supervisor

I was reminded of how parental experiences are very raw. Supervision often entails therapeutic use of self and transference or countertransference issues, and by exploring these feelings through the therapeutic application of STP, I facilitated insight into how parents may be feeling when their child comes to a therapist. The need to recognise our own triggers and bring them to supervision remained a foundation for growth and clinical decision-making.

For myself, I strongly believe that child treatment works best when parents are actively involved; being able to work with parents successfully is a crucial competency. I operate from a mindset where I "give my skills" to parents in the form of skill-sharing, coaching, and psychoeducation and often engage parents in structured approaches such as child-parent relationship therapy (Landreth & Bratton, 2019) and/or filial therapy (VanFleet, 1994). This particular supervision case offered me the opportunity to listen closely for what barriers may be present when parent disconnections or lack of engagement are happening and to explore the role of the supervisee in why and how this dynamic may be occurring. The bricks allowed the distance necessary to go back to previous painful moments and to facilitate the connections from the past to the current. In doing so, the therapist-in-training, parents, and the child client all benefit.

Case study #5: Parent group: military non-deployed parent psychoeducation group

The following case is a composite of a psychoeducational group experience with non-deployed parents of elementary school aged children in an active military community. This case study was chosen to illustrate the role of STP in working with groups. This case study precedes the formalisation of the STP process and aligns more directly with the LSP process. An example of this case study as it relates to implementing play therapy groups is reported in Peabody (2022).

Context

Military deployment is considered a type of ambiguous loss wrapped tightly around a cascading set of uncertain familial changes (Cohen-Konrad, 2013; Huebner et al., 2007). While many non-deployed partners demonstrate adaptability and resiliency, others may struggle with a range of emotions and difficulties consistent with anxiety, depression, or sleep disturbances (Kees & Rosenblum, 2015; Mansfield et al., 2010). Offering an experience of STP to the non-deployed parents is an example of mutual peer support and psychoeducation.

Challenge

The challenge involved a phased process over several weeks that included four of the seven traditional LSP applications: individual models and stories, shared models and stories, creating a landscape, and making connections (Kristiansen & Rasmussen, 2014).

Process

The goals in the initial weeks of the psychoeducation group were to familiarise the parents with norms, expectations, learning objectives, and a basic understanding of the STP process. As is typical in many LSP or STP experiences, the first builds allowed the parents to become familiar with the specialised LEGO® kit pieces and to become acquainted with the prompt-build-share process. The parents were given a series of prompts that challenged them to metaphorically represent a range of emotions related to military life and parenting. A psychological sense of safety was built from the very beginning through sensitive facilitation, navigating the validation of parental stories, and encouraging supportive responses amongst the other parents in the group.

Building upon the group's psychological safety for several weeks, parents built 3-D LEGO® models representing both the joys and tension of parenting during deployment (Figure 11.10). A continuum of emotionally laden stories and 3-D construction builds emerged. Stories of prideful belonging to the military community; coping under uncertainty; living through quasi-single parenthood; being both parental roles which brought conflicting emotions such as resentment and exhaustion. The parents built models and stories representing fatigue around the unrealistic need to be positive for their children. Others depicted how difficult living up to the military cultural messaging of "being emotionally strong" during deployment truly was. As the parents began to share their experiences and their vulnerabilities, they found each other's stories comforting. As the group continued to meet, I asked for the parents to construct LEGO® builds that centred on successful coping strategies, family values, dreams, and future aspirations. I added specialised connecting LEGO® chains, links, strings, and tubes and they physically connected their models to others with an explanation of why the connection resonated with them. Physically connecting one's own model to another's model elicited deep dialogue.

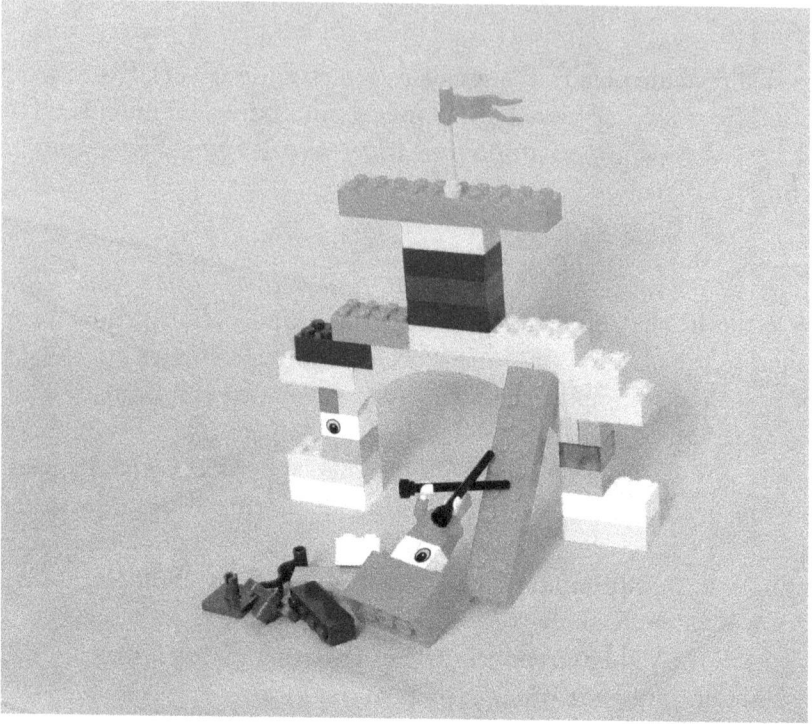

Figure 11.10 *A model depicting the emotions of pride and uncertainty.*

As the group came to a close, I intentionally offered prompts around endings and transitions. Living through deployments means goodbyes, transitions, and often relocation. Careful and respectful attention to endings and celebrations is important. The final prompt was to build a model representing the overall STP group experience. Brick models that symbolised giving and receiving support, play, comradery, and permission to break down the facade of "being strong all the time" all appeared in the final LEGO® builds. As I facilitated a process of closure and reflection, the parents shared insights, surprises, and experiences of validation that they were not alone amongst one another (Figure 11.11).

Insights of group members and facilitator

By externally using LEGO® bricks in a therapeutic application with topics related to the joys, frustrations, fears, and resiliency of parenting through military deployment, parents were offered a unique experience

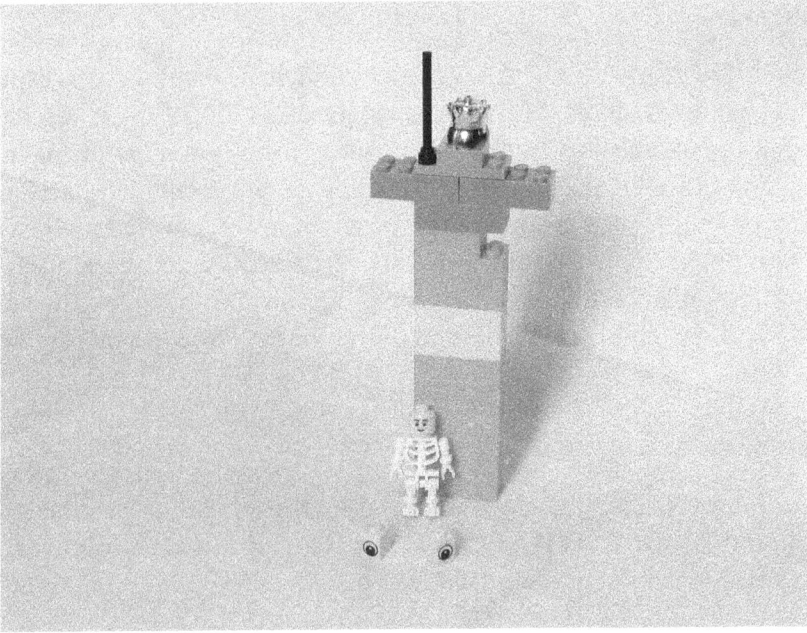

Figure 11.11 *Model demonstrating the experience of presenting a façade of always "being military strong" even during quasi-single parenthood.*

to symbolically express thoughts, feelings, and mutual support for one another. As the facilitator, watching the mutual support between the parents grow was rewarding and critically important for the needed social support. Military life is a chosen culture and hard to understand if one isn't experiencing it first-hand. To offer a space for relationships that provide a place for mutual sharing, laughter, learning and emotional sharing, and a space the parents began to look forward to each week was important. Several parents stayed connected after the group, and I believe the STP experience was the catalyst for those relationships to form.

Case study #6: Virtual group: building through a screen

In many ways, this case study highlights the context within which STP was initially conceived: supporting groups with specific mental health challenges. This case study was selected to highlight the experiences and potential for STP in virtual therapeutic contexts.

Context

During the height of the COVID-19 pandemic, many people experienced significant mental health challenges. This global event offered a unique opportunity to test many of our theories about implementing play-based LEGO® techniques in an online environment. This facilitator developed an 8-week group therapy program to be delivered in 90-minute sessions via an online platform. Six participants from three different countries initially self-selected for the program, and following the completion of the eight formal sessions, five continued to participate on a less formal basis.

Challenge

The primary challenge being addressed by these sessions was the stress presented by the COVID-19 challenge. Participants all acknowledged stress and anxiety as primary factors and so the program

Process

Throughout the eight 90-minute sessions, participants were asked to build representative models of their values, beliefs, and thought processes to help them to understand their anxiety or stress responses. Participants were also asked to build metaphorical models to help them envision goals and action-oriented statements for their futures. The eight sessions were organised in a progression from psychoeducation around stress, anxiety, and group play-therapy to examining self-beliefs and problematic patterns to living a valued life and building willingness. Participants were also given "homework" and asked to build and reflect upon models between the weekly sessions. Ultimately, the focus was on using LEGO® to allow participants to creatively imagine a different future and to make sense of their strategies for getting from their current reality of living with stress and anxiety to an imagined a future that may still include these challenges but was in some way "next level."

In week 7 of the program, participants were asked to combine several models from previous sessions and create their own values compass from the models, identifying their "true North" as well as any other models or values that provide them guidance. This challenge resonated with participants in a truly meaningful way; every participant shared images or videos of their compass with the group *before* the final session. Figure 11.12

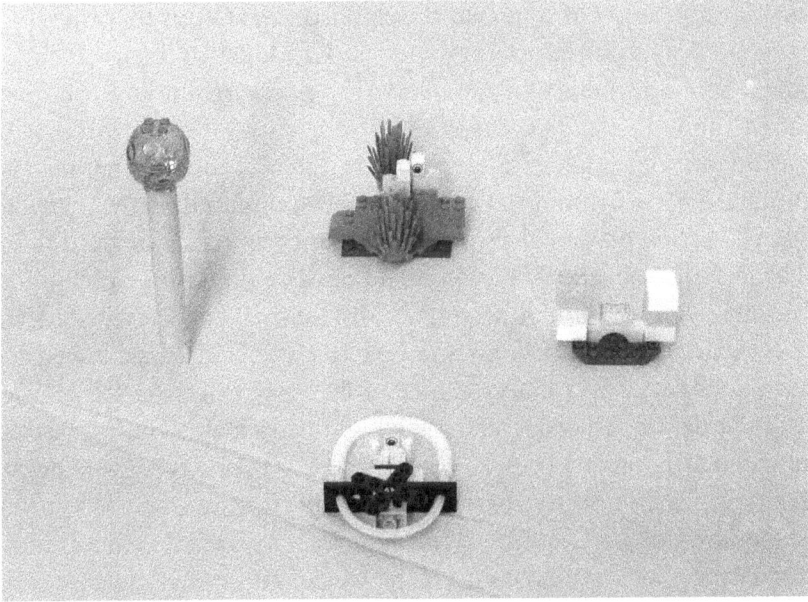

Figure 11.12 *Four LEGO® models organised in a compass pattern; growth (N), trust, (E), honesty (W), and adaptability (S).*

is one example of a values compass presented by one of the participants. The four compass points that this participant highlighted were growth (N), trust, (E), honesty (W), and adaptability (S). The model representing growth at the North compass point included mostly green and green and blue pieces and two eyes facing each other, speaking to the need for insight for this growth to occur. At the East point, the model contained mostly solid bricks, representing a need to protect the trust others place in the builder. At the South position, the adaptable model had movement, contained bendable pieces, and specifically included pink bricks, as the builder discussed her personal dislike for the colour pink. Finally, at the West position, the model for honesty included a transparent blue globe holding golden pieces, indicating a desire to rise above the fear and provide honesty for both the builder and others.

Insights

Participants
Following the 8 weeks, participants were asked for feedback regarding the program, what was valuable to them, and what they might change

about the experience if they had the opportunity. Given that these individuals were all LSP facilitators and used LEGO® in their practice of problem-solving, there was a consistent theme surrounding the investment in the emotional piece. With the focus on anxiety, there wasn't the avoidance of the feelings or emotions the way there sometimes is in traditional LSP workshops. Emotions were presented as the "problem to solve"; as one participant stated, "we went *there* and attended to it."

Participants collectively highlighted that, although they were building individually and the builds were very different, the stories shared were very similar and held common and relatable themes. This allowed for a common language and an experience of shared perspective. Camaraderie was clearly developed over the 8 weeks, and participants commented that their feeling of connection was deeper due to this shared experience and perspective. Although the participants came from diverse backgrounds (occupational therapy, business, academics, nursing, etc.), many stories held common metaphors. As is typical of the group therapy experience, participants found relief and solace in hearing each other's stories and their own stories reflected in others' words.

Finally, participants highlighted that, although the focus was pandemic-related stresses and anxiety, the conversations that were taking place by the end of the program were not really about the pandemic or other stresses that were occurring. Participants noted that the sharing extended beyond the LEGO®. For example, one participant wrote a song and shared a video, and another wrote a letter. The participants discussed the development of safety, which allowed the conversations to bleed into other places in their lives.

Facilitator

All participants completed all 8 weeks and did all the homework associated with the program (I can honestly say that, in my experience, I have never had 100% engagement in a group therapy program or a 100% completion rate of homework!). In fact, not only did they complete the homework, but participants indicated that the homework, which required them to share with other participants, served a stronger purpose in deepening the relationships and fortifying their connections. It is clear that this program fostered a sense of commitment, accountability, and belonging, and I believe that, because the participants experienced success, there was a strong desire to invest, both in themselves and the other participants.

For myself, as a facilitator, this 8-week program truly reinforced the need to get the questions or the prompt(s) to build right. Additionally, follow-up questions to the model cannot be scripted; genuine curiosity about the model(s) typically prompted the best questions and the best results for participants. Particularly in an online environment, I believe quiet facilitation is necessary; the facilitator cannot be distant and must be emotionally present. Additionally, I feel that co-creation is necessary for participants to engage; the facilitator must also be willing to offer vulnerability and authenticity if they expect those gifts from their participants. This also reminded me of the need for professionals to have a space to experience and process their own emotions (and not just in the context of supervision).

Although I was initially sceptical about the online nature, I recognise that virtual play-based work is not only possible but highly relevant and extremely valuable. At this particular time and place in history, virtual work highlighted that, while we were being isolated, we could still be in community.

Case study #7: Higher education: playful teaching and learning

Our final case study presents an application of STP to burgeoning therapists. Again, this case study precedes the formalisation of the STP approach, and so many of the reflections align with LSP as well.

Context

Adapting the use of LEGO® SERIOUS PLAY® (LSP) in higher education is well documented (James & Nerantzi, 2019). The growing number of publications across a variety of disciplines includes articles in business, leadership, nursing, engineering, occupational therapy, and counselling, to name a few (Dann, 2018; Dykes, 2018; Harn, 2017; Jensen et al., 2018; Kurkovsky, 2015; Nerantzi & James, 2019; Peabody & Noyes, 2017; Zenk et al., 2018). Each year, more articles are published as professors discover the power of this pedagogical approach.

The following case example is a sampling of how I designed a graduate-level play therapy theories course around STP to enhance knowledge integration and deepen student understanding and competence in communicating about play therapy theories, concepts, and definitions individually and collectively. I believe that learning itself is inextricably emotional, and learning to be a child therapist is a highly affective experience that continually challenges assumptions, values, ethical decisions, and practices. As such, using STP effectively provides students with tools to gain a better understanding of themselves and, in turn, aids in self-care and well being.

Challenge

The overall working assumption in using STP in a theories course was that personal and group reflections through LEGO® model construction could be a rich source of perceptual information to teach counselling theories and apply theory to practice. Borrowing on ideas of LSP in higher education, I wanted to foster a playful pedagogy to future play therapists, highlighting storytelling and metaphoric symbolism as a way to communicate and effect change.

Process

Each student was provided with a LSP starter kit for the week-long course, and the class size was small, allowing for full-group or small-group sharing. Each day the instructor would have the students build approximately three or four models to different prompts related to the content or personal reflections. Some of the prompts were a summary of learning prompts specific to theory or concepts discussed in the course. Other prompts were more reflective based in emotional content. Four of the five nights, homework was assigned to build a model that reflected a day's learning for them. This could be something that resonated with them positively or was a source of concern or tension. Examples of prompts given during the class:

- Build a model that represents a key concept from the "therapeutic powers of play" we discussed that is still unclear for you.
- Build a model that showcases two key concepts from the XXX theory of play therapy that aligns with your counselling values.
- Build a model of what counselling theory or theories we have explored this week that most closely aligns with how you view children and families make changes.
- Build a model that represents emotions that you experienced based on the video we just watched about aggression and limit setting in the playroom.

- Build a model that represents feelings/emotions you are experiencing after our role-play sessions.
- Build a model that addresses the "imposter syndrome" students have as they reflect on becoming a counsellor (Figure 11.13).
- Build a model that either excites/surprises or frustrates you about play therapy. You choose what you need today to express.

On the final afternoon of the course, we individually built our own definition of play therapy. Learning to describe play therapy to the public, including parents seeking treatment for their child, is a learned skill. Each student individually built their definition of play therapy and shared their model and definition. Next, individual models were then combined to create a communal "mega-story" of the definition of play therapy (Figure 11.14). Volunteers shared the mega-story out loud, ensuring the capture of the unique individual builds in the overall definition. Finally, we examined the definition of play therapy shared on day 1, with the communal build definition, to see how it compared. The group was then invited to explore adding, changing or keeping the model and their associated definition.

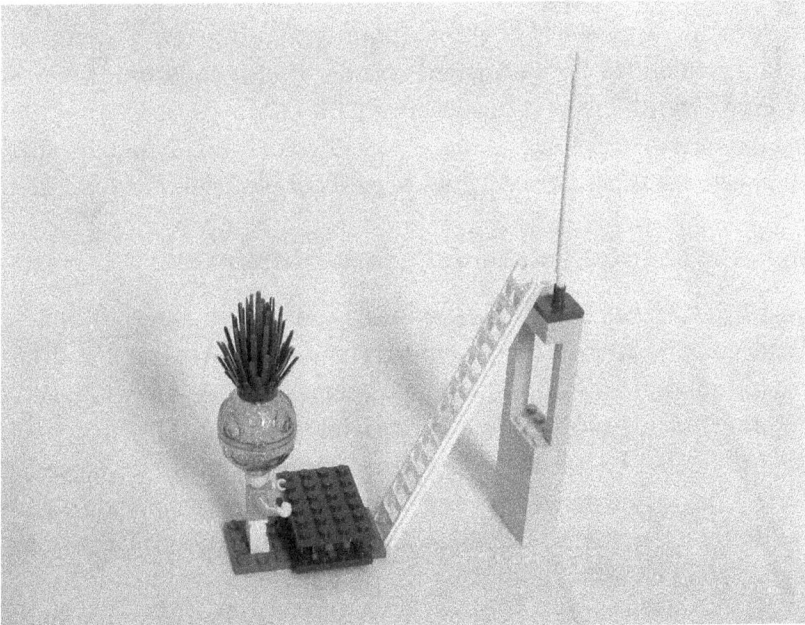

Figure 11.13 *A model illustrating imposter syndrome built by a student therapist.*

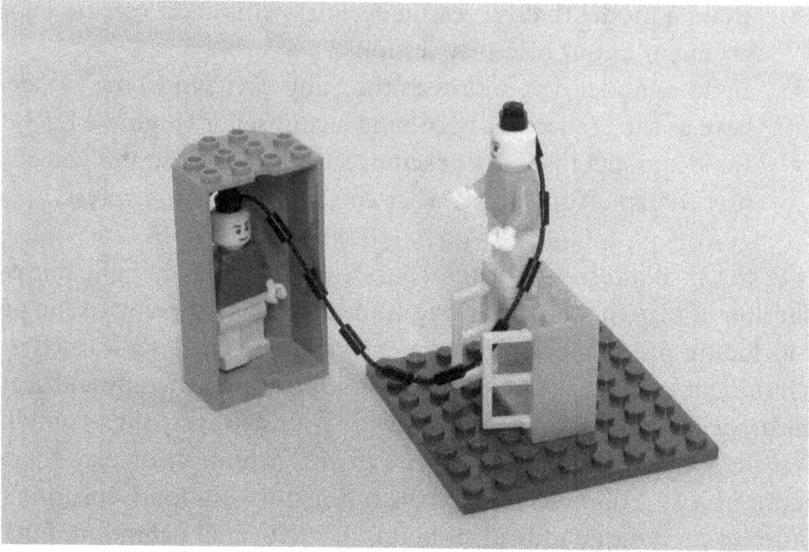

Figure 11.14 *A model demonstrating child development theories.*

For the last builds of the course, each student built two models. On one side was a representation of the "next steps" in their play therapy journey. The other side was an appreciation build reflective of the shared group experience. Students built future coursework, finding supervisors, speaking with their advisors about internship options. Appreciation builds included honouring the role of play for children, recognising their own playfulness, and diving deeply into themselves in a week-long course vs. a semester long course, the wisdom and vulnerability sharing of their classmates, and the positive playful course facilitation and design.

Insights of the students and the faculty member

Using LEGO® bricks in place of traditional journaling or reflective essays throughout the course was an immersion into visual and tangible instruction, hands-on thinking, perspective taking, listening, and the facilitated, safe expression of emotions while learning. This creative pedagogy proved to be a very positive and emotionally rich experience for the students, as evidenced by their course evaluations. Understanding play and its many therapeutic benefits is the foundation of becoming an effective child clinician, and using STP is a perfect marriage.

As the faculty member, I believe modelling play-based communication is essential for future play therapists. I firmly believe that the embodied hand-mind-feelings connection requires time for reflection and sharing. I believe that play therapists must enjoy the nuances of play and believe STP offers a structure – a pacing dynamic – that gives all students a voice. In this expressive experience, students experience a parallel experience of psychological safety in the classroom that I hope they can experience with future child clients in the safety of the playroom. Experiencing the therapeutic powers of play to express ideas, feelings, and future aspirations is vital to becoming a competent play therapist-in-training

Conclusion

We hope that it is evident from these case studies that the STP method is robust within multiple therapeutic contexts and settings. Our initial insights suggest that the method is effective for people of all ages and for individual and group therapeutic work. We have also found that the STP method has value in working both in-person and virtually. The aspect we think has significant power is the fun it creates through building; at times, participants can be overwhelmed by their stories, and the building seems to lighten the load and adds a sense of serious play and fun that helps them to move forward.

Additionally, we hope that, through the various cases, you, as the reader, can bear witness to how the nuanced questions interact, intersect, and shift the process. We also hope you better understand how inviting, holding, moving through, or around the edges of emotionally laden stories allows for change to take place. By metaphorically allowing you to sit alongside the case study narratives, you are offered insight into both the participant's process and the rare experience of what we as therapeutic facilitators were thinking and reflecting upon before, during, or after the STP experience.

We recognize that STP as a process, although robust, is still in its nascent stage, and there is significant room for growth. We have highlighted in the next chapter those "lessons learnt" in development of the process.

References

Brown, N., & Collins, J. (2018). Using LEGO® to understand emotion work in doctoral education. *International Journal of Management and Applied Research*, 5(4), 193–209. https://doi.org/10.18646/2056.54.18-014

Cohen-Konrad, S. (2013). *Child and family practice: A relational perspective*. Oxford Publishing.

Dann, S. (2018). Facilitating co-creation experience in the classroom with LEGO® SERIOUS PLAY®. *Australasian Marketing Journal, 26*(2), 121–131. https://doi.org/10.1016/j.ausmj.2018.05.013

Dowell, K. A., & Ogles, B. M. (2010). The effects of parent participation on child psychotherapy outcome: A meta-analytic review. *Journal of Clinical Child & Adolescent Psychology, 39*(2), 151–162. https://doi.org/10.1080/15374410903532585

Dykes, W. W. (2018). *Play well: Constructing creative confidence with LEGO® SERIOUS PLAY®* [Doctoral dissertation, Fielding Graduate University]. www.academia.edu/42964534/Play_Well_Constructing_Creative_Confidence_With_LEGO_Serious_Play?auto=download

Friedberg, R. D., & McClure, J. M. (2015). *Clinical practice of cognitive therapy with children and adolescents: The nuts and bolts* (2nd ed.). Guilford Press.

Harn, P. (2017). A preliminary study of the empowerment effects of strength-based LEGO® SERIOUS PLAY® on two Taiwanese adult survivors by earlier domestic violence. *Psychological Studies, 62*(2), 142–151. https://doi.org/10.1007/s12646-017-0400-3

Huebner, A. J., Mancini, J. A., Wilcox, R. M., Grass, S. R., & Grass, G. A. (2007). Parental deployment and youth in military families: Exploring uncertainty and ambiguous loss. *Family Relations, 56*(2), 112–122. https://doi.org/10.1111/j.1741-3729.2007.00445.x

James, A., & Nerantzi, C. (Eds.). (2019). *The power of play in higher education.* Springer. https://doi.org/10.1007/978-3-319-95780-7

Jensen, C. N., Seager, T. P., & Cook-Davis, A. (2018). LEGO® SERIOUS PLAY® in multidisciplinary student teams. *International Journal of Management and Applied Research, 5*(4), Article 4. https://doi.org/10.18646/2056.54.18-020

Kees, M., & Rosenblum, K. (2015). Evaluation of a psychological health and resilience intervention for military spouses: A pilot study. *Psychological Services, 12*(3), 222–230.

Kristiansen, P., & Rasmussen, R. (2014). *Building a better business using the LEGO® SERIOUS PLAY® method.* John Wiley & Sons.

Kurkovsky, S. (2015, June). Teaching software engineering with LEGO® SERIOUS PLAY®. *Proceedings of the 2015 ACM Conference on Innovation and Technology in Computer Science Education.* https://doi.org/10.1145/2729094.2742604

Landreth, G. L., & Bratton, S. (2019). *Child parent relationship therapy (CPRT): A 10-session filial therapy model.* Routledge.

Lin, Y.-W., & Bratton, S. C. (2015). A meta-analytic review of child-centered play therapy approaches. *Journal of Counseling & Development, 93*(1), 45–58. https://doi.org/10.1002/j.1556-6676.2015.00180.x

Mansfield, A. J., Kaufman, J. S., Marshall, S. W., Gaynes, B. N., Morrissey, J. P., & Engel, C. C. (2010). Deployment and the use of mental health services among U.S. army wives. *New England Journal of Medicine, 362*(2), 101–109. https://doi.org/10.1056/NEJMoa0900177

Nerantzi, C., & James, A. (2019). *LEGO® for university learning: Inspiring academic practice in higher education.* https://doi.org/10.5281/zenodo.2813448

Peabody, M. A. (2022). Constructing together: Therapeutic applications of LEGO® SERIOUS PLAY®. In C. Mellenthin, J. Stone, & R. J. Grant (Eds.), *Implementing play therapy with groups: Contemporary issues in practice* (pp. 15–25). Routledge.

Peabody, M. A., & Noyes, S. (2017). Reflective boot camp: Adapting LEGO® SERIOUS PLAY® in higher education. *Reflective Practice, 18*(2), 232–243. https://doi.org/10.1080/14623943.2016.1268117

Schaefer, C. E. (2003). *Play therapy with adults* (pp. xii, 392). John Wiley & Sons.

VanFleet, R. (1994). *Filial therapy: Strengthening parent-child relationships through play.* Professional Resource Press.

Watkins, C. E. (2020). Psychotherapy supervision: An ever-evolving signature pedagogy. *World Psychiatry, 19*(2), 244–245. https://doi.org/10.1002/wps.20747

Zenk, L., Hynek, N., Schreder, G., Zenk, A., Pausits, A., & Steiner, G. (2018). Designing innovation courses in higher education using LEGO® SERIOUS PLAY®. *International Journal of Management and Applied Research, 5*(4), 245–263. https://doi.org/10.18646/2056.54.18-019

CHAPTER 12
MORE THAN JUST INSTRUCTIONS AND MORE
THAN JUST BRICKS

Alec Hamilton, Mary Anne Peabody, and Kristen Klassen

When you first open a LEGO® kit and look at the myriad pieces, it is sometimes impossible to imagine what they will become. In some magical way, rigid, angular, and unicolour bricks are transformed to produce dynamic, fluid, vibrant representations of both the real and imaginary worlds. Somehow, 1 + 1 + 1 becomes 4.

In this chapter, we have pulled from our experience how we came to STP and what we have learnt along the journey. We work through both best practices that have worked for us and consistently bring positive results and lessons learnt through trial and error (i.e., those practices that, in our experience, do not bring about successful outcomes).

We return to our original lens of the biopsychosocial approach that guided the structure of our thinking and writing. We discuss the interconnections between the domains of the approach (biological, psychological, and social/environmental) and explore how it all comes together to become more than the sum of its parts. Each domain has a place in the STP process, working in a holistic and integrative way to create a transformative experience for therapeutic change.

Finally, the practitioner community and end-users are invited to contribute to the further development of STP.

DOI: 10.4324/9781003260424-13

Journey towards STP

Alec

One's journey towards something is often a journey away from something else. This is true of my journey towards using LEGO® in therapy. As a child, I was not a LEGO® person. I don't remember having LEGO® at all, nor was I attracted to it as an adolescent. I had not really thought about using it within my therapeutic practice until I was introduced to LEGO® SERIOUS PLAY® (LSP). I was completing my PhD and was very stuck interpreting the data visually. My partner is an LSP facilitator, and they had been, I felt in my stressed and overwhelmed state, badgering me to try LSP. However, I simply couldn't see how those childish coloured bricks could help me work through the complexity of my significant, academic, and scholarly work. My PhD was serious, meaningful, and vital for the world to read. It was definitely NOT about play and couldn't possibly be helped by a kid's toy. My journey towards Seriously Therapeutic Play (STP) was a journey away from the hassle of disagreeing with my partner and a desperate attempt to avoid being stuck, frustrated, and ready to give up.

My STP journey started when I gave in to being mature enough to play. I sat at our kitchen table with an LSP kit spread out in front of me and started to build what I thought my PhD was saying. I was still unconvinced that this would help, but I was now resigned to having a go. I started to build, and Anita was present with me but gave me the space to try and explain what I was building (Figure 12.1). Her calm and balanced manner was not the tone I deserved for all my complaints over the past weeks. About 10 minutes into the build, I was hit hard. We all know "aha" moments, but this just "aha"'d me to the core. These bloody bricks were starting to tell the story I had not been able to articulate. Elements suddenly started to literally emerge out of the table. My drawn models of circles and lines became alive and moving. I built, rebuilt, reviewed, and rebuilt again. All the while, Anita stayed with me as a quiet, calm presence, prompting and listening. There was a sense of excitement, my thoughts were clearer, and the model itself was much more complex – the 3-D aspect of the model I had not been able to see before.

My PhD model had grown in complexity and gave much greater depth and a richer sense of the relationships I was trying to present. I had been LSP'd. I also think now, in retrospect, that I had just experienced

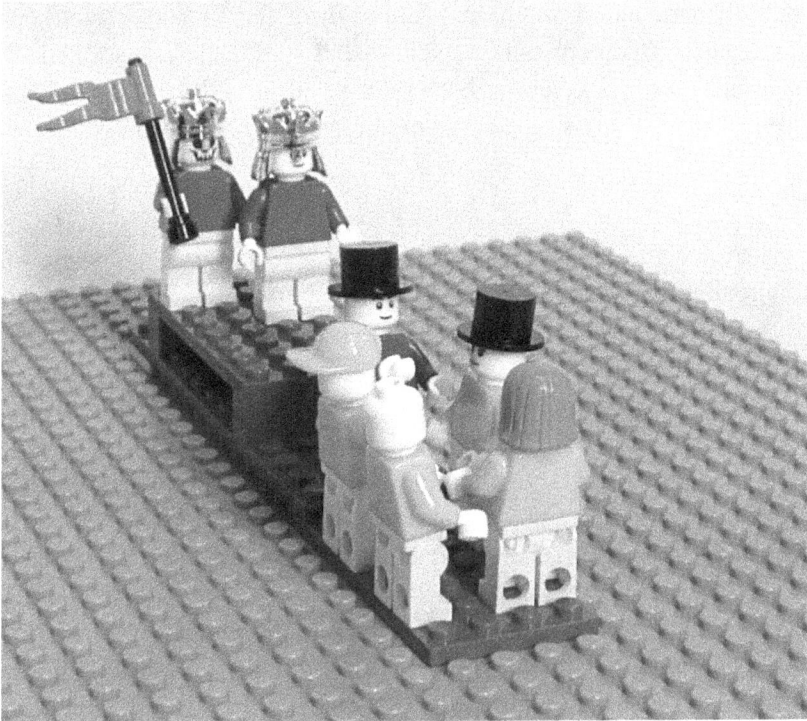

Figure 12.1 *The final LEGO® build developed for the PhD.*

my first sense of STP. Anita had used their skills as an LSP facilitator but had added to this their skills as a therapist. Anita recognised that there was a level of emotionality underlying the discussion that needed to be explored. This was not simply a series of strategies to work through to the next step in problem-solving. Anita needed to manage and facilitate my high levels of emotionality, allowing and pushing me to be present with my emotions and use them to build the metaphor I was constructing. After all, my PhD was about understanding presence within the context of therapy, and what I hadn't realised was that I needed someone's presence to help me shift my thinking. I needed her combined therapist and facilitator skills in directing and prompting my experience and understanding of the build.

Anita was intentional and stayed within the process in a way that helped me see anew and assisted me to then integrate my inner ponderings and conceptualisations via those childish colour bricks. The symbolism held within the 3-D LEGO® model and its various components more fully articulated anything I had seen or felt before. Together, we had seriously therapeutically played with LEGO®. I was hooked. Not long after, I was lucky enough to be trained in LSP by my co-author, Kristen. I have been using STP in my practice ever since.

Mary Anne

My journey with LSP and STP started many years ago, but maybe I just didn't realise it. Interestingly, as a child, I didn't have LEGO® bricks to play with, and in fact, I didn't purchase any for my own children. Even as I became a children's play therapist, I had shelves of wooden and soft blocks that were a popular staple in the playroom; however, I only had a small bucket of LEGO® bricks available in the playroom. It truly wasn't until I was trained in LSP that I realised the expressive and narrative power of the small coloured bricks and began to use them more intentionally in a more directive approach with some child clients, but most of my LEGO® interactions were with adults.

As my play therapy practice changed and I became a full-time professor, I was compelled to bring my knowledge and passion for the therapeutic powers of play to my adult students (Figure 12.2). I began to explore the literature to see how other professors were using LSP in their classrooms and wanted to add to that field of knowledge and practice. I saw such great potential and eventually signed up for the LSP training to deepen my understanding and experience the methodology myself. As I sat through the LSP training, I was reminded of all my sandtray experiences, yet sand and LEGO® as tactile sensory experiences are totally different. The ability to "build and create" elements; to take apart, change, or rebuild the model as needed; and the 3-D capabilities created many "aha" moments. While I have always been attracted to and utilised metaphors, symbolism, and object play, the feel of the bricks, the story sharing, and a structured methodology for communication had points of both connection and productive friction for me. The questions were many. How can I bring this methodology to my students, to my research agenda, and to my scholarship around teaching and learning?

Two pivotal points occurred next. I felt a strong need to meet with individuals already using LSP in ways that I wanted to in my classroom and practice. I wanted to learn from their expertise. When I was in London, I set up a meeting with Alison James, a LSP facilitator who uses the methodology with her collegiate students to help them become deep

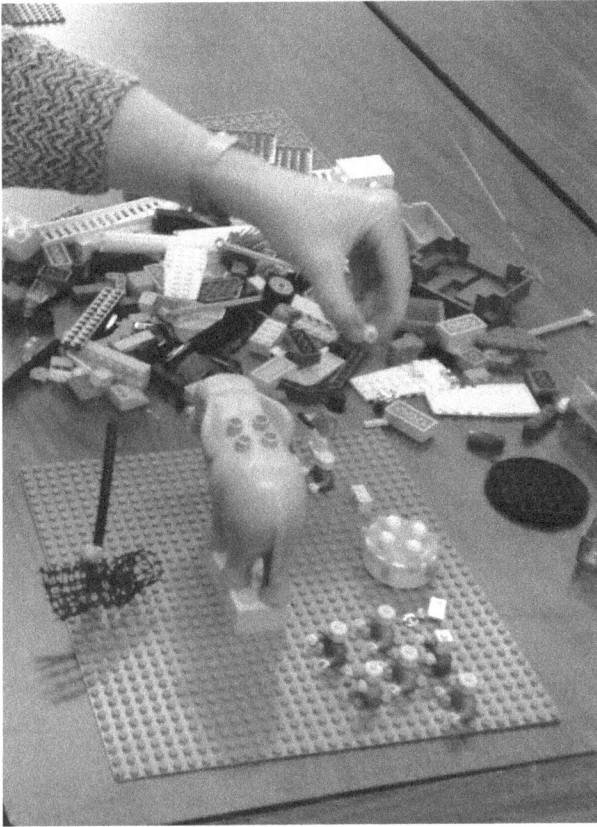

Figure 12.2 *A 3-D construction emerging in the context of higher education.*

reflective thinkers. As reflective practice is a key competency for training mental health professionals, I viewed LSP as a vehicle to teach and extend reflective practice skills. I emailed Alison to see if we could meet, and she graciously accepted. I was thrilled to talk with her about both reflective practice and how she was using the bricks to create powerful and transformative learning experiences for her students. I returned back to the classroom and offered a variety of focussed LSP-adapted experiences with my students. The more I offered the methodology, the more I witnessed the power inherent in the bricks and the facilitation of the process to bring forth emotions and stories. I was intrigued.

The second pivotal point came when I discovered Kristen, my co-author. Kristen is a trainer of facilitators in LSP, therapist, business entrepreneur, and academic. Better yet, she was scheduled to do a LSP training in Boston, just 2 hours away from me! I sent her an email and asked if we could meet for dinner while she was in Boston. Between laughter and many slices of pizza, I knew I had met someone who shared the potency of the affective side of the LSP experience. She understood the potential and power of the facilitated process and had a vision for therapeutic possibilities by not only mental health professionals but others in helping related fields. If my flame of excitement had been smouldering before, Kristen added both oxygen and fuel to the mix, igniting my creativity and motivation. We talked for hours about possibilities I might explore with an upcoming sabbatical and I began formulating my potential agenda.

I continued to use what I termed an "adaptation of LSP" in various settings: my courses in social and behavioural sciences, adult training workshops, clinical play therapy supervision, parent consultation, and parent psychoeducational groups. What I didn't realise was I was experimenting with what would later become STP. Soon, Kristen was offering her therapeutic application of the LSP model in an 8-week virtual course (due to the pandemic), and I signed up to be a participant. Another powerful experience that solidified my convictions around the seriously therapeutic play model with LEGO®. From that experience came several discussions and connections that Kristen had with Alec, and the idea of writing a book proposal together was born.

Along with the many positive "aha" moments along the journey, there were moments that caused me to pause. While I valued and understood the therapeutic powers of play and, specifically, the importance of object and symbolic play, I soon realised not all adults share this knowledge or are ready to engage in it. In fact, while the novelty of the bricks as communication is typically met with excitement and openness to playfully experiment, there have been times when a small number of adults participated with hesitation or scepticism. Some struggled with the methodology's symbolic or metaphoric nature, while others struggled with the actual building of LEGO® brick construction, resulting in minor frustration. Over time, I have experimented with how to address this early in the beginning minutes of using STP. I start with an invitational *permission to play* invitation and always honour the importance of the traditional LSP *warm-up skill builds* to set the psychologically safe tone, further discussed in our lessons learnt.

Kristen

My journey was, in many ways, the complete opposite of both Alec's and Mary Anne's; I was enamoured with LEGO® as a child and built continuously throughout my adolescence. LEGO® was my number one item on every Christmas and birthday wishlist. I built structured kits from instructions and MOCs (My Own Creations), and I played imaginatively with what I built. Building with LEGO® was not only a creative and imaginative endeavour, it was also a peaceful and mindful experience for me. I only slowed my playing when I left home for University, and it became impractical for me to transport my expansive (and still growing) LEGO® collection through ever-changing dorm rooms, apartments, and across multiple degrees in multiple cities.

My exposure to LEGO® SERIOUS PLAY® (LSP) came during my first master's degree, and I felt an immediate connection with the method. In addition to rekindling my love of the bricks, the approach resonated with me and my core beliefs about play. After being trained, I started my side hustle, Brickstorming, and began using the LSP method in the traditional contexts for which it was designed: solving corporate problems and organisational challenges. I experimented with the method in research contexts as well as with children but did not genuinely venture into the affective or emotional applications.

My transition to STP came with my progression from LSP facilitator to Trainer of Facilitators (ToF). At the time, I had recently completed my PhD and was working in a research capacity within a mental health clinic. I was also working to complete my play therapy certification. I was fortunate to be mentored in my journey to ToF by one of the original developers of the LSP method. I spent time observing his craft and saw that, while the purpose of LSP is not therapy, there was therapeutic change happening; there were opportunities to deepen and widen the emotional context, allowing for corrective emotional experiences. The training in LSP is not designed to accommodate these experiences, but I could see the potential in the core process. After certifying as a ToF, I began working on what I termed "LSP for therapeutic applications" (LSPTA).

The final push to STP came in the form of the pandemic; my friend and fellow facilitator (Ana) reached out to me to ask if I would be willing to put together a version of my LSPTA for an online group, supporting people as they were coping with the fallout from the pandemic (Figure 12.3). This shift in intention was the final catalyst for me. I invested deeply in the emotional potential and created an 8-week therapeutic program focussed on stress and anxiety. I purposefully selected questions and building prompts that explored the affective experience and did not seek to solve any particular problem. The program was a

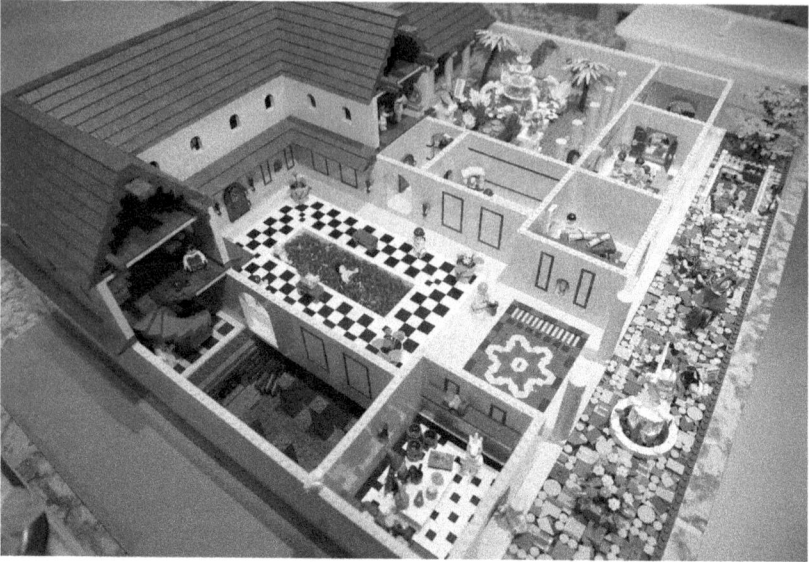

Figure 12.3 *A Roman villa designed and built in 2016, around the same time as the transition to STP began.*

success by every measurement; all six participants completed all 8 weeks of the program (including their "homework" builds completed outside of the group sessions), and five of them continued to meet on an informal basis for almost a year after the conclusion of the program. I continued to offer the program with additional groups and through this process was reconnected with Alec and Mary Anne.

I found kindred spirits in my co-authors; and I do not use that term lightly. I believe that the term describes people who share a deep connection, an unspoken understanding, and a bond that transcends words and logic. Alec and Mary Anne bring out the best in me and have been amazing collaborators throughout this process of delineating what STP is and what it is not.

Lessons learnt

One premise that emerged for us all during or from our LSP training is that the old analogy reverberates in our discussions: "you can take the girl out of Texas, but you can't take Texas out of the girl." We share the simple belief you can take the therapist out of the therapeutic context, but you cannot take the therapist out of the person. All three of us have developed a style of applying LSP ideas and processes to therapy, arriving at this juncture because we saw a usefulness in the method and how it might be successfully adapted to our contexts. The following are some of the goal posts or mile markers that have helped us stay on track in developing and using STP.

Lesson 1: Get hands on bricks ASAP

One of the first facilitative lessons we learnt over the years is to let the participants *get their hands on the bricks* sooner than later. Mary Anne commented that, early in her journey, she presented an entire lengthy presentation about the process, underlying theories, and the research ("yes, as an academic, this is hard to let go of"). She quickly discovered that it was the experiential, hands-on sharing where the transformations took place. Now, after a brief introduction, she gets the participants building! Alec noted that, when working with children, he found that "they couldn't keep their hands off the LEGO®" once they saw it and were given permission to play. We still all get all the important information shared throughout our time together. It is simply spread out throughout the experience rather than front-loaded.

Lesson 2: Give permission to play

When the learning process is more geared toward STP outcomes, another lesson may need to be addressed. Some participants may struggle with how a serious issue (chronic illness, family disruption, caregiving, or stress) can be paired with a toy. This stems from their belief that *play is a fun experience*, and therefore, there is potential for cognitive dissonance. A *"permission-to-play"* invitation is key to mitigating this and establishing psychological safety. Mary Anne highlighted that, in her experience, the invitation itself is most effective when it speaks (briefly) to the knowledge around the neuroscience of object play across the lifespan and the emotional wellness benefits associated with adult play. Speaking to the connotation of the word *play* and matching it with other words, such as creativity, innovation, and divergent thinking can often help to dispel any initial scepticism. As well, differentiating between play as an enjoyable, intrinsically motivated activity and serious play that invokes conscious reflection on the activity itself in a way that directly connects to real-life issues and concerns can reassure potential participants of the value in the experience. Depending on the audience, the *permission-to-play* message may need to be adapted with a more academic and research-based slant or simply an invitation to try, experiment, explore, and be curious. We especially like the challenge that many LSP facilitators put forth: "Are you mature enough to play?".

Lesson 3: Lean in to the affective side

In traditional serious play interventions, there is a desire to lean away from the affective responses, whereas in STP, active observation of verbal and nonverbal communication leads to affect recognition. In other words, we believe that the facilitator should focus on the nonverbal communication and emotionally laden words that a participant may use. While we know that, if it is therapeutically important, the client will revisit the issue until it is resolved, we don't want to miss this opportunity to ask for further elaboration on the model or to connect participants' stories to one another and to deepen the possibilities for self-awareness. We stay with the participant in the affective experience, or in a group situation connecting and sharing the affective pieces of the participants' stories with one another.

Lesson 4: Pay attention to pacing and structure

The STP-facilitated process also honours the importance of pacing and structure, providing an environment that includes individual discoveries and collaborative activities. The group dynamic rules of LSP and STP – where *everyone participates equally* – is a bit foreign to typical therapy group rules, so navigating this is the facilitator's responsibility. Skilful facilitation requires a level of flexibility in order to explore the unforeseen openings and space for the sensitive issues that arise. Individuals inherently know the level of distress their system can tolerate, so allowing enough time for self-titration is key. Additionally, we must be able to draw out quieter voices while simultaneously adhering to the time needed to ensure the steps of the core process are all achieved. Therefore, it is a vital lesson to pay attention to pacing and time constraints to ensure there is enough time for reflection.

Lesson 5: Establish physical and psychological safety

Early in our STP journeys, we recognised the importance of the physical environment and room set-up to psychological safety, and this should be carefully thought through. This obviously depends on the time and space available, which we do not always have control over, but it can impact successful facilitation. In group settings, it is vital to focus on an intentional creation of a space where participants can see each other's models and clearly hear one another. When working one-to-one, a space needs to be created that allows for serious play that is age appropriate. Some adults love sitting on the floor to build others do not. We need to help them be comfortable choosing what is right for them.

Additionally, we have found that our positioning with respect to the individual, model, and group is essential; it is key in an STP context that the physical space does not take on an investigation or assessment dynamic – i.e., where the facilitator and participant are located across from each other. This type of dynamic amplifies power imbalances, reduces psychological safety, and moves participants towards work rather than play. We are also very careful in taking time to reflect on what worked well in terms of space and what has been less valuable with the participants so we can improve with each facilitated opportunity and each context.

Summary of lessons learnt

We have all learnt a process that is strategic and intentional. As mentioned earlier, we clearly differentiate between an enjoyable, intrinsically motivated activity that is play and "serious play" that invokes conscious reflection on the activity itself in a way that directly connects to real-life issues and concerns. Both are useful in the spaces we share with our participants but have very different purposes and contexts. We think this book captures the next step in our collective journeys in developing our understanding of the importance of having clearly articulated structures and processes in strategically using LEGO® but also an awareness of having a serious approach to working with the narratives and emotionality of therapy. We are adamant in our belief that STP, at its core, is *not* simply playing with bricks but a way to consciously and ethically use the metaphors and symbolism that emerges in building with LEGO® in therapy to aid our participants.

Returning to the biopsychosocial lens

As our book concludes, we revisit the biopsychosocial lens used to organise our thinking and sharing. We stated in the introductory chapter that we divided the book into four parts; the first three chapters focussed on the biological components, the middle three chapters focussed on the psychological components, the next four focussed on the social components, and the final two chapters on how we use the approach in a more integrated nature. The domains are not discrete, linear, or sequential; rather, they are interrelated.

As you have read the chapters, you will have noticed the interrelatedness of the domains. We believe that the overall STP process, while based in the biological, psychological, and social/emotional research, is best described as a fluid, dynamic, and interconnected experience. We view the facilitator as operating in each domain simultaneously, traversing across the them in a holistic manner where biological, psychological, and social processes blend and overlap synergistically. Synergy is combining two or more entities that result in a greater sum than the individual efforts can achieve. Applying a holistic and synergistic mindset offers the STP facilitator a way of conceptualising how the domains are metaphorically "playing with one another" in a meaningful and integrative way.

Just as a pile of bricks are individual parts, it is typically not until the bricks are connected to one another that a three-dimensional model with an associated story and metaphor begins to take form. As such, each of the biopsychosocial domains are central and essential to the creation of therapeutic change for our participants. When the individual parts are taken together, it is then that the STP journey truly begins!

Where are you?

We finish with an invitation to you, the reader. We truly hope to create a community of practice; thinking about your own journey, where are you? How are you using LEGO® in your therapeutic practice, and what would you like to know more about? As noted in the introduction, this book is our guidebook to "why" we believe the therapeutic use of LEGO® is both valuable and an excellent resource in any therapist/facilitator's tool bag or tickle trunk. It is our foundational piece to STP. However, we recognise that we are influenced by our own lens and that not all relevant theories and foundational pieces have been investigated. Perhaps there are pieces from your perspective that would deepen the understanding of this process?

Following this, we also plan to produce the playbook on the "how" of STP in practice, which will provide the reader with practical solutions and supporting materials. We'd like to know what would facilitate this learning for you and where are your current stuck points? In essence, what guideposts do you need to make effective use of this technique? We can't wait to continue this journey with you!

INDEX